Management of GERD: Looking with 2020 Vision

Editor

KENNETH J. CHANG

GASTROINTESTINAL ENDOSCOPY CLINICS OF NORTH AMERICA

www.giendo.theclinics.com

Consulting Editor
CHARLES J. LIGHTDALE

April 2020 • Volume 30 • Number 2

ELSEVIER

1600 John F. Kennedy Boulevard • Suite 1800 • Philadelphia, Pennsylvania, 19103-2899

http://www.theclinics.com

**GASTROINTESTINAL ENDOSCOPY CLINICS OF NORTH AMERICA Volume 30, Number 2
April 2020 ISSN 1052-5157, ISBN-13: 978-0-323-75464-4**

Editor: Kerry Holland
Developmental Editor: Donald Mumford

Gastrointestinal Endoscopy Clinics of North America (ISSN 1052-5157) is published quarterly by Elsevier Inc., 360 Park Avenue South, New York, NY 10010-1710. Months of issue are January, April, July, and October. Business and Editorial Offices: 1600 John F. Kennedy Blvd., Suite 1800, Philadelphia, PA, 19103-2899. Periodicals postage paid at New York, NY and additional mailing offices. Subscription prices are $359.00 per year for US individuals, $655.00 per year for US institutions, $100.00 per year for US and Canadian students/residents, $399.00 per year for Canadian individuals, $774.00 per year for Canadian institutions, $476.00 per year for international individuals, $774.00 per year for international institutions, and $245.00 per year for international students/residents. To receive student/resident rate, orders must be accompanied by name of affiliated institution, date of term, and the *signature* of program/residency coordinator on institution letterhead. Orders will be billed at individual rate until proof of status is received. Foreign air speed delivery is included in all *Clinics* subscription prices. All prices are subject to change without notice. **POSTMASTER:** Send address change to *Gastrointestinal Endoscopy Clinics of North America*, Elsevier Health Sciences Division, Subscription Customer Service, 3251 Riverport Lane, Maryland Heights, MO 63043. **Customer Service: 1-800-654-2452 (US). From outside the United States, call 1-314-447-8871. Fax: 1-314-447-8029. E-mail: JournalsCustomerService-usa@elsevier.com (for print support) or JournalsOnlineSupport-usa@elsevier.com (for online support).**

Reprints. For copies of 100 or more, of articles in this publication, please contact the Commercial Reprints Department, Elsevier Inc., 360 Park Avenue South, New York, NY 10010-1710. Tel. 212-633-3874; Fax: 212-633-3820; E-mail: reprints@elsevier.com.

Gastrointestinal Endoscopy Clinics of North America is covered in *Excerpta Medica, MEDLINE/PubMed (Index Medicus), and MEDLINE/MEDLARS.*

Contributors

CONSULTING EDITOR

CHARLES J. LIGHTDALE, MD
Professor of Medicine, Division of Digestive and Liver Diseases, Columbia University Medical Center, New York, New York, USA

EDITOR

KENNETH J. CHANG, MD, FASGE, FACG, AGAF, FJGES
Professor and Chief, Gastroenterology and Hepatology Division, Executive Director, H.H. Chao Comprehensive Digestive Disease Center, Vincent and Anna Kong Chair of GI Endoscopic Oncology, University of California, Irvine Medical Center, University of California, Irvine, Orange, California, USA

AUTHORS

CAROLINE M. BARRETT, MD
Department of Internal Medicine, Vanderbilt University Medical Center, Nashville, Tennessee, USA

REGINALD BELL, MD, FACS
Institute of Esophageal and Reflux Surgery, Englewood, Colorado, USA

PETROS C. BENIAS, MD
Director of Endoscopic Surgery, Assistant Professor of Medicine, Division of Gastroenterology, North Shore-Long Island Jewish Medical Center, Donald and Barbara Zucker School of Medicine at Hofstra/Northwell, Northwell Health System, Manhasset, New York, USA

NIKOLAI BILDZUKEWICZ, MD, FACS
Assistant Professor of Clinical Surgery, Associate Program Director for the General Surgery Residency and The Advanced GI/MIS Fellowship, Keck Medical Center of USC, Los Angeles, California, USA

KENNETH J. CHANG, MD, FASGE, FACG, AGAF, FJGES
Professor and Chief, Gastroenterology and Hepatology Division, Executive Director, H.H. Chao Comprehensive Digestive Disease Center, Vincent and Anna Kong Chair of GI Endoscopic Oncology, University of California, Irvine Medical Center, University of California, Irvine, Orange, California, USA

STEVEN R. DeMEESTER, MD
Thoracic and Foregut Surgery, General and Minimally Invasive Surgery, The Oregon Clinic, Portland, Oregon, USA

COLIN DUNN, MD
PGY4 Resident, General Surgery, Rutgers New Jersey Medical School, Newark, New Jersey, USA

TYRALEE GOO, MD
Tibor Rubin Veterans' Affairs Medical Center Long Beach, Long Beach, California, USA

PHILIP O. KATZ, MD
Professor of Medicine, Division of Gastroenterology and Hepatology, Weill Cornell Medicine, New York, New York, USA

ROBERT H. LEE, MD, MAS
H.H. Chao Comprehensive Digestive Disease Center, University of California, Irvine, Irvine, California, USA; Tibor Rubin Veterans' Affairs Medical Center Long Beach, Long Beach, California, USA

JOHN LIPHAM, MD, FACS
Chief of Division of Upper GI and General Surgery, President of the American Foregut Society, James and Pamela Muzzy Endowed Chair, Upper GI Cancer, Keck Medical Center of USC, Los Angeles, California, USA

RACHEL NIEC, MD, PhD
Fellow in Gastroenterology, Division of Gastroenterology and Hepatology, Weill Cornell Medicine, New York, New York, USA

JOHN E. PANDOLFINO, MD, MSCI
Division of Gastroenterology and Hepatology, Northwestern University Feinberg School of Medicine, Chicago, Illinois, USA

DHYANESH PATEL, MD
Division of Gastroenterology, Hepatology and Nutrition, Vanderbilt University Medical Center, Nashville, Tennessee, USA

KARA L. RAPHAEL, MD
Division of Gastroenterology, North Shore-Long Island Jewish Medical Center, Donald and Barbara Zucker School of Medicine at Hofstra/Northwell, Northwell Health System, Manhasset, New York, USA

JASON B. SAMARASENA, MD
Associate Professor of Medicine, University of California, Irvine, Orange, California, USA

FELICE SCHNOLL-SUSSMAN, MD
Professor of Clinical Medicine, Division of Gastroenterology and Hepatology, Weill Cornell Medicine, New York, New York, USA

PIOTR SOWA, MD
University of California, Irvine, Orange, California, USA

STUART JON SPECHLER, MD
Division of Gastroenterology, Center for Esophageal Diseases, Baylor University Medical Center at Dallas, The Center for Esophageal Research, Baylor Scott & White Research Institute, Dallas, Texas, USA

MICHAEL F. VAEZI, MD, PhD
Division of Gastroenterology, Hepatology and Nutrition, Vanderbilt University Medical Center, Nashville, Tennessee, USA

PATRICK WALSH, MD
Division of Gastroenterology, St Vincent's Northside Medical Centre, Brisbane, Australia

RENA YADLAPATI, MD, MSHS
Division of Gastroenterology, University of California, San Diego, La Jolla, California, USA

ROBIN A. ZACHARIAH, MD
H.H. Chao Comprehensive Digestive Disease Center, University of California Irvine, Irvine, California, USA

Contents

Gastroesophageal reflux (GER) describes a process in which gastric contents travel retrograde into the esophagus. GER can be either a physiologic phenomenon that occurs in asymptomatic individuals or can potentially cause symptoms. When the latter occurs, this represents GER disease (GERD). The process by which GER transforms into GERD begins at the esophagogastric junction. Impaired clearance of the refluxate also contributes to GERD. Reflux causes degradation of esophageal mucosal defense. The refluxate triggers sensory afferents leading to symptom generation.

Patients with gastroesophageal reflux disease (GERD) present with heterogeneous symptoms, response to treatment, and physiologic profiles, requiring distinct and personalized management. This article provides a stepwise framework to phenotype GERD beginning with (1) characterization of symptom profile and response to acid suppression; (2) endoscopic evaluation of mucosal and anatomic integrity; (3) ambulatory reflux monitoring to characterize reflux burden and sensitivity; and (4) esophageal physiologic testing to assess gastroesophageal reflux mechanism and effectors of reflux clearance, and evaluate for alternate causes.

Proton pump inhibitors (PPIs) continue to be the medication of choice for treatment of acid-related disease, with few if any overt side effects seen with daily use. They are often prescribed empirically, often in high doses and with many patients being treated with multiple PPIs without an objective diagnosis. Therefore, they are believed to be overprescribed and used without indication. In this article we discuss the appropriate clinical indications for PPIs, review in detail the major associated adverse events, and put in perspective key issues in balancing benefits and risk of this exceptional (and safe) class of drug.

> Gastroesophageal reflux disease (GERD) is the most frequent outpatient
> diagnosis in the United States. There has been significant development
> in the endoscopic treatment of GERD, with several devices that have
> reached the market. One of the endoscopic devices for the management
> of GERD in the United States is the Stretta system. This procedure uses
> radiofrequency energy, which is applied to the muscles of the lower
> esophageal sphincter and the gastric cardia resulting in an improvement
> of reflux symptoms. This review evaluates the most recent data on the ef-
> ficacy, mechanisms of action, and safety of this procedure.

> GERD is a spectrum disorder, and treatment should be individualized to
> the patient's anatomic alterations. Trans-oral incisionless fundoplication
> (TIF 2.0) is an endoscopic procedure which reduces EGJ distensibility,
> thereby decreasing tLESRs, and also creates a 3-cm high pressure zone
> at the distal esophagus in the configuration of a flap valve. As it produces
> a partial fundoplication with a controlled valve diameter, gas can still
> escape from the stomach, minimizing the side-effect of gas-bloat. Herein
> we discuss the rationale, mechanism of action, patient selection, step-by-
> step procedure, safety and efficacy data, it's use with concomitant laparo-
> scopic hernia repair, and future emerging indications.

 Video content accompanies this article at http://www.giendo.
theclinics.com.

> Minimally invasive endoscopic antireflux therapies are critical for bridging
> the gap between medical and surgical treatments for gastroesophageal
> reflux disease (GERD). Although multiple endoscopic devices have been
> developed, perhaps some of the most exciting options that are currently
> evolving are the full-thickness suturing techniques using widely available
> and low-cost platforms. Full-thickness endoscopic suturing can allow for
> a highly durable recreation of the anatomic and functional components
> of a lower esophageal sphincter, which are deficient in patients with
> GERD. Proper patient selection, endoscopic hiatal hernia evaluation,
> and standardized suturing methods are necessary to ensure success of
> endoscopic suturing for antireflux therapy.

> Antireflux surgery is challenging, and has become even more challenging
> with the introduction of alternative endoscopic and laparoscopic options
> for patients with gastroesophageal reflux disease (GERD). The Nissen

fundoplication remains the gold standard for the durable relief of GERD symptoms and esophagitis. All antireflux procedures have a failure rate, and it is important to minimize factors that are associated with failure. The selection of patients for antireflux surgery as well as the choice of the procedure requires a thorough understanding of esophageal physiology and the pros and cons of various options.

GASTROINTESTINAL ENDOSCOPY CLINICS OF NORTH AMERICA

FORTHCOMING ISSUES

July 2020
Colorectal Cancer Screening
Douglas K. Rex, *Editor*

October 2020
Endoscopy in the Era of Antibiotic Resistant Bacteria
Jacques Van Dam, *Editor*

January 2021
Advances in Barrett's Esophagus
Sachin Wani, *Editor*

RECENT ISSUES

January 2020
Endoscopic Closures
Roy Soetikno and Tonya Kaltenbach, *Editors*

October 2019
Colonoscopic Polypectomy
Douglas K. Rex, *Editor*

July 2019
Inflammatory Bowel Disease
Simon Lichtiger, *Editor*

RELATED CLINICS SERIES

Gastroenterology Clinics
Clinics in Liver Disease

THE CLINICS ARE AVAILABLE ONLINE!
Access your subscription at:
www.theclinics.com

Foreword

Gastroesophageal Reflux Disease: Changing the Conversation

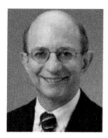

Charles J. Lightdale, MD
Consulting Editor

Every once in a while, a field that has felt static for decades begins to move. Gastro-esophageal reflux disease (GERD) is in one of those times. GERD is a big modern prob-lem with estimates of significant GERD in some 30 million in the United States. For a long while, treatment has boiled down to 2 options: the pill (proton pump inhibitors, PPIs) or the knife (laparoscopic fundoplication). There is no doubt that these treat-ments benefit a majority of patients suffering from GERD but have also left many dissatisfied. A combination of factors seems to be involved in creating this movement. There have been new insights into the pathophysiology of GERD and a clear percep-tion that all GERD patients are not alike and need to be identified with more precision and managed differently.

GERD is a chronic disease. Low-acid diets and weight loss can be very helpful but difficult to achieve and maintain. PPIs, considered for years to be among the safest of pharmaceuticals, were associated in long-term observational studies with a multitude of serious side effects, which have not been confirmed in more rigorous studies except for a higher risk of enteric infections. Yet, PPIs are not successful for symptom relief in some patients, and younger patients are concerned with taking them indefinitely. Laparoscopic fundoplication also helps most patients, but can cause unpleasant side effects, and also can loosen with time, requiring repeat operations or a return to PPIs.

Ken Chang, an internationally renowned leader in gastroenterology and gastrointes-tinal endoscopy, is the editor of this issue of *Gastrointestinal Endoscopy Clinics of North America* focused on the evolving management of GERD. He has developed a remarkable collection of topics authored by a terrific group of experts. The articles on pathophysiology and personalized approaches, a review of PPIs, extraesophageal GERD, and laryngopharyngeal reflux, refractory GERD, and functional heartburn will appeal to gastroenterologists and esophagologists. Articles on emerging endoscopic

Gastrointest Endoscopy Clin N Am 30 (2020) xi–xii
https://doi.org/10.1016/j.giec.2020.02.001
1052-5157/20/© 2020 Published by Elsevier Inc.

therapies for GERD, including Stretta and transoral incisionless fundoplication, are certain to interest interventional endoscopists and foregut surgeons, who will also gain much from the reviews of fundoplication and magnetic lower-esophageal sphincter augmentation. The field of GERD is moving. Read this outstanding issue in its entirety. It will change the conversation about GERD.

Charles J. Lightdale, MD
Department of Medicine
Columbia University Medical Center
161 Fort Washington Avenue
New York, NY 10032, USA

E-mail address:
CJL18@columbia.edu

Preface

The New Landscape of Gastroesophageal Reflux Disease Management: 2020 and Beyond

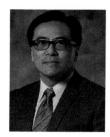

Kenneth J. Chang, MD, FASGE, FACG, AGAF, FJGES
Editor

The landscape of gastroesophageal reflux disease (GERD) management is changing, in a good way. Several key forces have converged (**Box 1**), propelling us to see GERD with a new perspective. One of these forces is the expanding role of the interventional gastrointestinal endoscopist in foregut diseases, including GERD, Barrett's and early esophageal cancer, achalasia, Zenker diverticulum, early gastric cancer, gastric outlet obstruction, and obesity. Accordingly, when tapped by Dr Lightdale to be the editor of this issue devoted to GERD management, I had the privilege of assembling some of the

---

Box 1
Key converging factors or forces propelling a new perspective on gastroesophageal reflux disease management

1. The prevalence of GERD, Barrett's, and esophageal adenocarcinoma appears to be rising.

2. Many patients are either not satisfied with their GERD symptom control or wish to come off their PPI medications.

3. Patients and surgeons are shying away from Nissen fundoplication due to side effects of gas and bloating, thus energizing innovation of new techniques and devices.

4. The pathophysiology and anatomical alterations of GERD are better understood; hence, targeted, personalized treatment strategies, including endoscopic approaches, have emerged.

5. The GERD treatment team has expanded to include primary care, advanced practice provider, gastroenterologist, esophagologist, interventional endoscopist, surgeon, and psychologist.

Gastrointest Endoscopy Clin N Am 30 (2020) xiii–xiv
https://doi.org/10.1016/j.giec.2020.01.001
1052-5157/20/© 2020 Published by Elsevier Inc.

giendo.theclinics.com

top GERD authorities, including esophagologists, interventional endoscopists, and foregut surgeons. The other key forces or factors are highlighted throughout the 10 articles of this issue, culminating in a new 2020 approach to GERD management and treatment. In "Mechanism and Pathophysiology of Gastroesophageal Reflux Disease," the authors bring to light that the lower esophageal sphincter (LES), while a very important antireflux barrier, is not the only factor and possibly may not be the most crucial factor. The hitherto underappreciated diaphragmatic crus (namely, the right crus) has only recently been recognized for its antireflux function, which extends well beyond the passive role of preventing the stomach from herniating into the chest. Its dynamic and complex "sling" action on the gastroesophageal junction is now understood to be critical in GERD pathophysiology. In addition, as is highlighted in several of the articles, the LES is in reality not just in the esophagus. The inner circular muscles of the distal esophagus are actually in continuity and become the sling fibers of the proximal stomach. This important fact helps us to understand how and why antireflux procedures (including laparoscopic and endoscopic) may be working to reduce the number and amount of reflux episodes. GERD is now appreciated to be a spectrum disorder, with different degrees of anatomical alterations occurring in each individual patient. In "Personalized Approach in the Workup and Management of Gastroesophageal Reflux Disease," the authors use a clever analogy to the card game, Texas Hold'em, to present a logical step-wise approach in identifying the individual patient's GERD phenotype, which will lead to the most efficient and effective treatment strategy. "Proton Pump Inhibitors: The Good, Bad, and Ugly" equips the practitioner with the current expert consensus regarding the safety and side effects of proton pump inhibitor (PPI) medications. "Nonablative Radiofrequency Treatment for Gastroesophageal Reflux Disease (Stretta)" and "Transoral Incisionless Fundoplication" go into great depth to summarize the indications, mechanism of action, and outcomes of the 2 Food and Drug Administration–approved endoscopic antireflux procedures. "Innovations in Endoscopic Therapy for Gastroesophageal Reflux Disease" discusses emerging endoscopic approaches to GERD that leverage the gastric side (sling fibers) of the LES. "Laparoscopic Hernia Repair and Fundoplication for Gastroesophageal Reflux Disease" provides historical context and practical guiding principles to antireflux surgery. "Magnetic Sphincter Augmentation for Gastroesophageal Reflux Disease" shows how magnetic sphincter augmentation has revitalized antireflux surgery with a technically easier and more standardized operation. "Refractory Gastroesophageal Reflux Disease and Functional Heartburn" takes a deep dive into reflux hypersensitivity and functional heartburn, while "Laryngopharyngeal Reflux and Atypical Gastroesophageal Reflux Disease" gives a fresh perspective to extraesophageal reflux syndromes, including novel biomarkers and mucosal integrity testing, and exciting new treatment developments.

Kenneth J. Chang, MD, FASGE, FACG, AGAF, FJGES
H.H. Chao Comprehensive Digestive Disease Center
University of California, Irvine
101 The City Drive
Orange, CA 92868, USA

E-mail address:
kchang@uci.edu

Mechanism and Pathophysiology of Gastroesophageal Reflux Disease

Robin A. Zachariah, MD[a], Tyralee Goo, MD[b], Robert H. Lee, MD, MAS[a,b],*

KEYWORDS

- Gastroesophageal reflux disease • Esophagogastric junction • Hiatal hernia
- Crural diaphragm

KEY POINTS

- A complex sequence translates gastroesophageal reflux into gastroesophageal reflux disease (GERD).
- Disruption of the antireflux barrier is the first step.
- Impaired reflux clearance contributes to GERD.
- Reflux leads to degradation of esophageal mucosal defenses.
- Activation of sensory afferents depends on refluxate features and sensitization.

INTRODUCTION

A distinction needs to be made between gastroesophageal reflux (GER) and reflux leading to symptoms or disease (GER disease[GERD]). GERD is defined as a condition in which reflux leads to "troublesome symptoms and/or complications."[1] In contrast, GER can be a physiologic phenomenon that occurs in asymptomatic individuals. The process by which GER leads to GERD consists of a sequence of events spanning the esophagogastric junction (EGJ), the esophageal body, and the central nervous system.

ESOPHAGOGASTRIC JUNCTION IN HEALTH

The antireflux barrier at the EGJ consists of the lower esophageal sphincter (LES), and the crural diaphragm (CD)[2] These superimposed structures constitute the antireflux barrier. Muscle fibers in the LES assume an incomplete C shape, forming clasp fibers

[a] H.H. Chao Comprehensive Digestive Disease Center, 333 City Boulevard West, Suite 400, Room 459, Orange, CA 92868, USA; [b] Tibor Rubin Veterans' Affairs Medical Center, 5901 E. Seventh Street, Long Beach, CA 90822, USA
* Corresponding author. H.H. Chao Comprehensive Digestive Disease Center, 333 City Boulevard West, Suite 400, Room 459, Orange, CA 92868.
E-mail address: rlee8@uci.edu

Gastrointest Endoscopy Clin N Am 30 (2020) 209–226
https://doi.org/10.1016/j.giec.2019.12.001
1052-5157/20/Published by Elsevier Inc.
giendo.theclinics.com

that surround each other and interact with gastric oblique or sling fibers (**Fig. 1**).[3] It has long been observed that the LES pressure profile is asymmetric, with LES peak pressures correlating with the maximum muscle thickness found on the greater curve of the stomach where the gastric sling fibers have the greatest density.[4]

The portion of the right crus of the CD through which the esophagus passes constitutes the external part of the antireflux barrier. Much like the LES, the pressure profile of the CD is asymmetric, with inspiration producing a more pronounced increase in EGJ pressure toward the greater curve of the stomach.[5] The CD produces a pinch-cock effect on the LES, with contraction during normal inspiration producing an increase of 10 to 20 mm Hg in LES pressure (LESP).[6] Using this salutary effect, Eherer and colleagues[7] trained patients with GERD in abdominal breathing techniques designed to augment CD function. With this training, the treated group had improvements in GERD-related quality-of-life scores and acid exposure times.[7]

ESOPHAGOGASTRIC JUNCTION IN GASTROESOPHAGEAL REFLUX DISEASE
Lower Esophageal Sphincter Integrity

GER occurs when intragastric pressure (IGP) exceeds LESP.[8] Hypotensive LES has been found to be associated with GERD dating back to the 1970s.[9] With the advent of high-resolution esophageal manometry (HRM), quantitative metrics have also pointed to impaired LES barrier function in GERD. Nicodeme and colleagues[10] quantified the contractile vigor of the LES using the EGJ contractile integral (CI) (**Fig. 2**). Using this parameter, studies have shown that patients with GERD have lower EGJ-CI values compared with normal subjects.[10–13] Despite these observations, a minority of patients with GERD have hypotensive LES.[14,15] Consequently, hypotensive LES cannot be the sole mechanism for GERD.

Transient Lower Esophageal Sphincter Relaxation

Transient lower esophageal sphincter relaxation (TLESR) was initially identified by Dent[16] as inappropriate LES relaxation lasting 5–30 seconds and that had a stronger

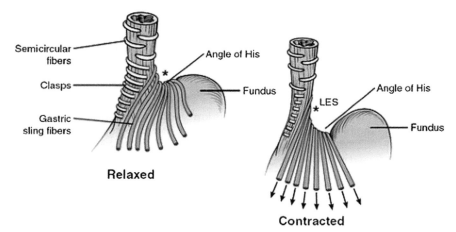

Fig. 1. LES fibers form an incomplete C shape that interfaces with gastric sling fibers. With contraction of the gastric fibers, the angle between the distal LES and the gastric fundus (angle of His) narrows.* Location of the LES in the relaxed state. (*From* Lerut T, Coosemans W, Decaluwe H, et al. The anatomy of the esophagus 2016. Available at: https://basicmedicalkey.com/the-anatomy-of-the-esophagus/. Accessed August 29, 2019, with permission.)

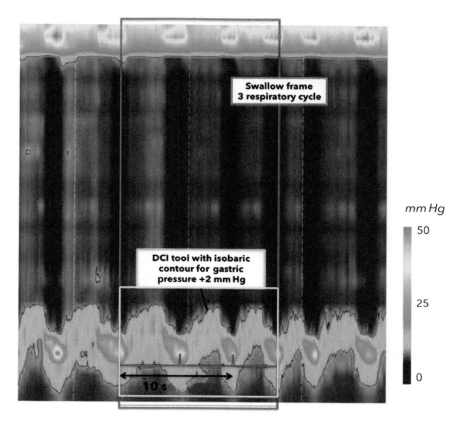

Fig. 2. EGJ-CI. On HRM, the isobaric contour is set to highlight the EGJ at a minimum of the gastric pressure +2 mm Hg. The smart mouse tool is used to measure the CI over 3 respiratory cycles. The CI is then divided by the time. DCI, distal contractile integral. (*From* Nicodeme, F., et al., Quantifying esophagogastric junction contractility with a novel HRM topographic metric, the EGJ-Contractile Integral: normative values and preliminary evaluation in PPI non-responders. Neurogastroenterol Motil, 2014. 26(3): p. 353-60, with permission.)

correlation with GER than low LESP. The modern definition of TLESR finds the following hallmarks: (1) CD inhibition, (2) absence of swallowing within 4 seconds of LES relaxation, (3) LES relaxation of greater than 10 seconds.[17]

Along with a transient decrease in LES contractility, other events occur with TLESRs. TLESRs are accompanied by axial shortening of the distal esophagus followed by a common cavity phenomenon marked by equalization of esophageal and IGP (**Fig. 3**),[18] which is followed by a positive pressure gradient in which IGP exceeds EGJ pressure.[18] It is also postulated that longitudinal muscle (LM) contraction triggers shortening of the esophagus, which produces axial strain on the LES leading to TLESR.[19,20] Furthermore, the degree of CD inhibition during TLESRs has been found to be directly correlated to the decrease in LESP.[21]

TLESR triggers include pharyngeal intubation, meal ingestion, upright posture, smoking, hyperglycemia, and intake of poorly digested carbohydrates.[22-27] Gastric distension, whether by air or meals, is a well-known trigger for TLESRs, producing a

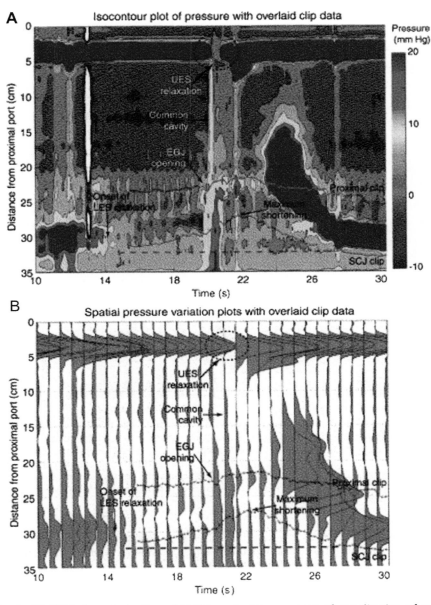

Fig. 3. (*A*) HRM characterization of TLESR marked by presence of equalization of pressures (common cavity) and EGJ opening. (*B*) HRM findings with overlay of fluoroscopy showing that these events occur in conjunction with esophageal shortening. UES, upper esophageal sphincter. (*From* Pandolfino, J.E., et al., Transient lower esophageal sphincter relaxations and reflux: mechanistic analysis using concurrent fluoroscopy and high-resolution manometry. Gastroenterology, 2006. 131(6): p. 1725-33, with permission.)

4-fold increase in the rate of TLESRs.[28] With meal ingestion, gastric accommodation typically offsets the change in IGP, which should limit the impact on TLESRs.[29] In conditions such as functional dyspepsia (FD) and gastroparesis in which gastric accommodation is impaired, meal intake can have a more profound impact on the frequency of TLESRs. Pauwels and colleagues[30] used an HRM-impedance catheter to measure IGP and found that restricted gastric accommodation quantified by a smaller change in IGP resulting in an increase in TLESRs after meal intake. This link between impaired gastric accommodation and TLESRs may also explain why up to 50% of patients with FD and 8% to 20% with gastroparesis have pathologic GERD.[31,32]

Since the 1980s, TLESRs have largely replaced hypotensive LES as the most widely accepted mechanism for GERD. In patients with esophagitis, 60% to 70% of TLESRs occur with acid reflux, compared with just 40% to 50% in controls.[33] Furthermore, TLESRs have been found to explain most daytime reflux episodes.[34] GERD treatments also decrease the frequency of TLESRs. Baclofen, a GABA-B receptor agonist, has been found to decrease TLESR frequency and CD inhibition.[35] Similarly, fundoplication has been found to produce a 50% reduction in TLESRs compared with baseline.[36]

Hiatal Hernia

With the movement of TLESRs to the forefront in the 1980s, the role of hiatal hernia (HH) became remarkably diminished. However, more recently it has again taken its rightful place in the understanding of reflux. At the turn of the century, Jones and colleagues[37] highlighted that HH was the most powerful predictor of esophagitis. Van Herwaarden and colleagues[38] found that patients with GERD with and without HH had the same frequency of TLESRs but that the HH group had twice the amount of acid exposure. Furthermore, 50% to 58% of patients with HH have visible esophagitis, compared with 3% to 7% of patients without HH.[39]

One of the obvious mechanisms underlying the relationship between HH and GERD is the separation of the CD and LES. The use of HRM has defined 3 distinct EGJ subtypes based on the CD-LES distance (**Fig. 4**).[40] Pandolfino and colleagues[41] found that EGJ type III, which had the greatest degree of separation, also had the lowest level of inspiratory augmentation of EGJ pressure. Furthermore, 37 out of 39 subjects with inspiratory augmentations of less than or equal to zero had pathologic reflux disease.[41] Several studies have also shown an association between EGJ type III and more significant levels of acid exposure.[10]

The presence of an HH contributes to GER through multiple mechanisms. Kahrilas and colleagues[42] found that HH status was the most powerful predictor of TLESR frequency. The interplay between HH and increased EGJ compliance is another mechanism. Pandolfino and colleagues[43] measured EGJ compliance using a hydrostat applying the law of Laplace to calculate the EGJ cross-sectional area (CSA) based on the known intrabag pressure and the degree of EGJ opening using fluoroscopy. EGJ opening occurred at pressures of less than 0 mm Hg only in subjects with GERD with HH compared with those without HH and controls. The GERD with HH group also had the most profound change in EGJ opening at any given pressure.[43] Recently, the functional lumen imaging probe (FLIP) has allowed easier measurement of EGJ distensibility and CSA (**Fig. 5**).[44] Kwiatek and colleagues[45] showed that distensibility was 2 to 3 times greater in patients with GERD compared with controls.

HH also promotes reflux through the acid pocket. The acid pocket refers to an area distal to the LES where acidity exceeds what is seen elsewhere in the esophagus or

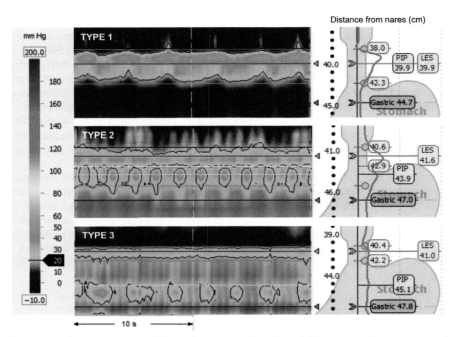

Fig. 4. HRM characterization of the EGJ. Type 1, the LES and CD are superimposed; type 2, LES and CD separation less than 3 cm apart; type 3, LES and CD 3 cm or more apart. (*From* Gyawali, C.P., et al., Classification of esophageal motor findings in gastro-esophageal reflux disease: Conclusions from an international consensus group. Neurogastroenterol Motil, 2017. 29(12), with permission.)

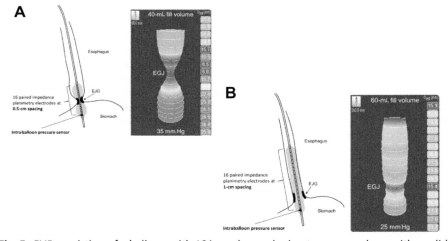

Fig. 5. FLIP consisting of a balloon with 16 impedance planimetry sensors along with a solid-state pressure sensor to measure intraballoon pressure. When the balloon is filled with saline, voltage can be calculated using Ohm's law. Because the CSA is proportional to the voltage, CSA values for esophageal lumen are calculated. (*A*) Patient with achalasia with noncompliant EGJ. (*B*) Patient with GERD with overly compliant EGJ. (*From* Carlson, D.A., Functional lumen imaging probe: The FLIP side of esophageal disease. Curr Opin Gastroenterol, 2016. 32(4): p. 310-8. Figure used with permission from the Esophageal Center at Northwestern.)

the stomach within 10 to 15 minutes of a meal.[46,47] The length of the acid pocket is longer in patients with GERD than in controls.[48,49] Furthermore, the longest zones of acidity occur in subjects with GERD with larger HHs.[48] Beaumont and colleagues[50] found that 77% of TLESRs in patients with large HHs and 54% of TLESRs with small HHs occurred when the acid pocket was located within the hiatus or above the diaphragm. Treatment with proton pump inhibitors (PPIs), baclofen, and raft-forming alginates all promote downward positioning of the acid pocket with resulting decreases in reflux.[51–55]

In addition, HH has a deleterious impact on reflux clearance. Sloan and Kahrilas[56] found that only 32% of swallows cleared the esophagus without retrograde flow in patients with nonreducing HH compared with 66% in those with reducible HH. Furthermore, in the nonreducible HH group, most incomplete emptying occurred because of retrograde flow from the hernia into the esophagus.[56]

Gastroesophageal Flap Valve

The sling fibers extending from the EGJ toward the greater curve of the stomach create a flap valve orientation in which distension of the gastric fundus leads to extrinsic compression on the distal esophagus.[2] The flap valve can be easily assessed during upper endoscopy using the Hill grade classification system, with a looser valve seen in Hill grade type IV (**Fig. 6**).[57] Patients with GERD have wider (more obtuse) insertion angles than controls, which resulted in a greater degree of EGJ opening and a larger number of reflux events.[58]

ACID PENETRATION OF ESOPHAGEAL MUCOSAL DEFENSE

The current GERD paradigm suggests that the acid directly erodes the esophageal mucosa (**Fig. 7**).[59] Once mucosal defenses are degraded, H^+ penetrates the submucosal layer, causing cell death and triggering an inflammatory response.[60] According to the paradigm, the easiest pathway for acid lies in the intercellular

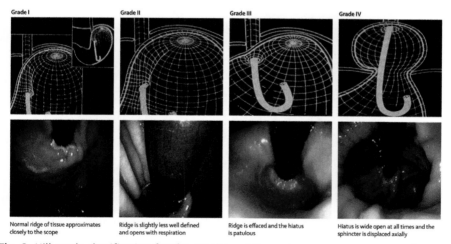

Grade I	Grade II	Grade III	Grade IV
Normal ridge of tissue approximates closely to the scope	Ridge is slightly less well defined and opens with respiration	Ridge is effaced and the hiatus is patulous	Hiatus is wide open at all times and the sphincter is displaced axially

Fig. 6. Hill grade classification for the esophageal flap valve as seen on upper endoscopy. Reprinted with permission from Elsevier [Bredenoord, A.J., J.E. Pandolfino, and A.J. Smout, Gastro-oesophageal reflux disease. Lancet, 2013. 381(9881): p. 1933-42].

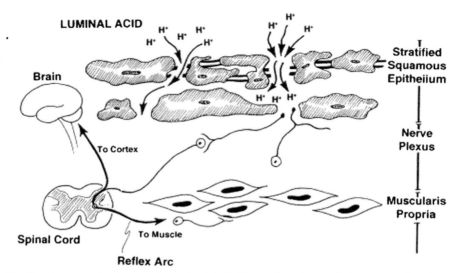

Fig. 7. H$^+$ penetrates the esophageal epithelial layer along intercellular spaces after degradation of glycoproteins. Dilated intercellular spaces (DISs) allow entry of H$^+$ into the submucosa to interact with sensory afferents triggering reflux symptoms. (*From* Barlow, W.J. and R.C. Orlando, The pathogenesis of heartburn in nonerosive reflux disease: a unifying hypothesis. Gastroenterology, 2005. 128(3): p. 771-8, with permission.)

spaces, which are protected by proteins such as claudins, occludins, and E-cadherin.[61,62] It is postulated that acid causes direct damage to these proteins, producing a greater diameter between cells in the form of dilated intercellular spaces (DISs) (**Fig. 8**).[63,64] In humans, DIS is found in 68.2% to 83% of patients

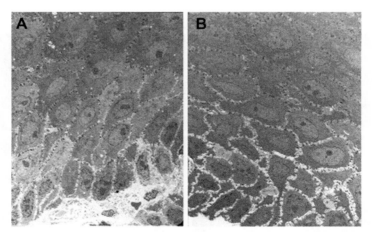

Fig. 8. Electron microscopy of esophageal epithelium. (*A*) Normal control with tight junctions between epithelial cells. (*B*) Patients with nonerosive reflux disease showing DISs. (*From* van Malenstein, H., R. Farre, and D. Sifrim, Esophageal dilated intercellular spaces (DIS) and nonerosive reflux disease. Am J Gastroenterol, 2008. 103(4): p. 1021-8, with permission.)

with nonerosive reflux disease (NERD), and 48% to 100% of those with erosive esophagitis (EE).[64] Indirect assessment for DIS has been proposed using baseline impedance (BI) measured by pH multichannel intraluminal impedance (MII). Using this metric, several studies have found that BI is significantly lower in patients with pathologic acid exposure.[65,66] Using a cutoff of less than 2100 Ω, Kandulski and colleagues[67] found that BI identified subjects with GERD and inversely correlated with DIS measurements.

More recently, Souza and colleagues[68] challenged this traditional paradigm, suggesting that the primary mode of injury is mediated by T lymphocytes. Among patients with GERD who discontinued PPIs 2 weeks before endoscopic biopsy, they found an increase in lymphocyte levels along with DIS in areas that were without surface erosions.[69] Specimens also stained positive for hypoxia-inducible factor (HIF) 2α, a proinflammatory cytokine that is induced by bile salts.[70] Under this alternative paradigm, acid and bile salts enhance stabilization of HIF-2α, leading to increases in levels of T-cell chemokines that promote esophagitis **(Fig. 9)**.[70]

IMPAIRED CLEARANCE OF THE REFLUXATE

Impaired peristalsis has long been associated with GERD. Manometry studies have shown lower contraction amplitudes in patients with EE compared with normal controls.[71–73] However, the process of clearing the refluxate is more complex than simply measuring manometric values. First, distension of the esophageal lumen by the refluxate causes a reflex mediated by stretch receptors in the esophageal wall,

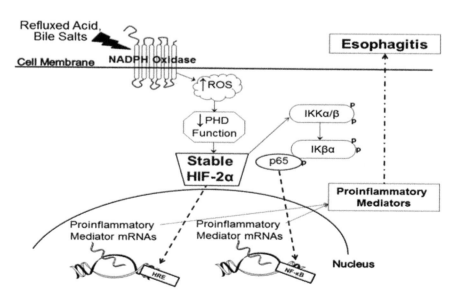

Fig. 9. Alternative mechanism to esophagitis. Bile salts stabilize HIF-2α, which results in T cell–mediated inflammation. IK, kappa kinase; IKK, I kappa kinase; mRNA, messenger RNA; NADPH, nicotinamide adenine dinucleotide phosphate, reduced form; NF, nuclear factor; PHD, prolyl hydroxylases; ROS, reactive oxygen species. (*From* Huo, X., et al., Hypoxia-inducible factor-2alpha plays a role in mediating oesophagitis in GORD. Gut, 2017. 66(9): p. 1542-1554, with permission.)

leading to secondary peristalsis and volume clearance.[74] However, even with volume clearance, there is often no change in acidity. In contrast, swallow-induced peristalsis (primary peristalsis) with ingestion of bicarbonate-containing saliva produces chemical clearance and pH normalization.[74]

The relationship between impaired primary peristalsis and GERD is highlighted by pH-MII studies. Frazzoni and colleagues[75] characterized the occurrence of chemical clearance by a swallowing episode that occurred within 30 seconds of reflux as a postreflux swallow-induced peristaltic wave (PSPW) (**Fig. 10**). A PSPW index was calculated based on the number of reflux episodes followed by a PSPW divided by the number of reflux events. The investigators found that the PSPW index was significantly lower in patients with pathologic esophageal acid.[75] A PSPW index with a cut-off of 61% also had the optimal receiver operating curve in predicting pathologic reflux.[76]

Along with primary peristalsis, secondary peristalsis is also impaired. Schoeman and Holloway[77] found that the success rate for eliciting a secondary peristaltic response was 0% among patients with GERD versus 30% to 50% in normal controls. More recently, Carlson and colleagues[78] used FLIP to identify repetitive anterograde contractions (RACs) as secondary peristaltic events in reaction to luminal distension (**Fig. 11**). Subjects without RACs had higher levels of esophageal acid.

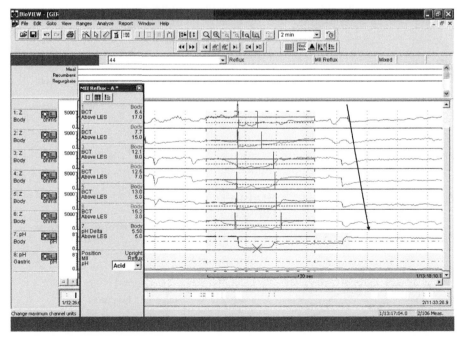

Fig. 10. pH-MII tracing in which a weakly acid reflux event is followed by a PSPW (*arrow*). PSPW is defined as an antegrade 50% decrease in impedance from baseline occurring within 30 seconds of reflux. (*From* Frazzoni M, Savarino E, de Bortoli N, et al. Analyses of the post-reflux swallow-induced peristaltic wave index and nocturnal baseline impedance parameters increase the diagnostic yield of patients with reflux disease. Clin Gastroenterol Hepatol 2016;14(1):40–6, with permission.)

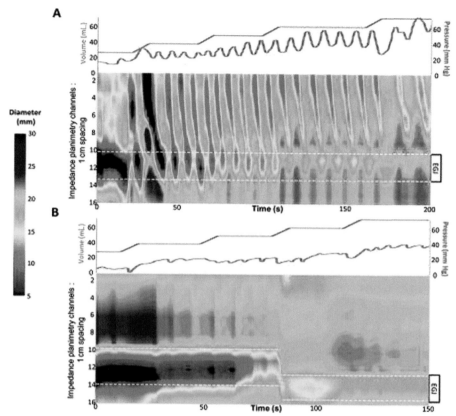

Fig. 11. FLIP topography in response to balloon distension. (*A*) Distension results in antero-grade contractions with acid exposure time (AET) of 4.9%. (*B*) No significant contractility seen in the esophagus in patient with AET of 29%. (*From* Carlson, D.A., et al., The relation-ship between esophageal acid exposure and the esophageal response to volumetric disten-tion. Neurogastroenterol Motil, 2018. 30(3), with permission.)

SYMPTOM GENERATION IN GASTROESOPHAGEAL REFLUX DISEASE

Once the refluxate is able to degrade mucosal defenses, reflux is then able to trigger symptoms. However, symptom generation is complex and much remains unknown about how signals are translated into sensations of heartburn. The apparent paradox of patients with Barrett's esophagus having few symptoms compared with patients with functional heartburn who have profound sensitivity points to there being multiple factors in the process of symptom generation.

Transient Receptor Potential Vanilloid-1

Transient receptor potential vanilloid-1 (TRPV1) receptors are calcium-permeable cation channels that are present on esophageal sensory afferents.[79] TRPV1 activa-tion occurs with exposure to heat and H^+; a decrease to a pH of 5 to 6; and capsa-icin, the key ingredient in chili peppers.[80] With activation, TRPV1 allows the passage of Ca and Na ions, leading to nerve depolarization.[81]

TRPV-1 may represent the primary afferent pathway for reflux symptoms. TRPV-1 expression is upregulated in patients with both EE and NERD (**Fig. 12**).[82,83] The potential role of TPRV1 activation in inducing GERD symptoms was highlighted in a study in which submucosal injection of capsaicin and not acid triggered severe sensations of heartburn and chest pain in healthy volunteers.[84]

Factors Determining Reflux Perception

pH-MII studies have found that more precipitous decreases in pH, proximal extent, delayed volume clearance, impaired acid clearance, and the presence of gas are all associated with symptom perception.[85–89] The presence of acid in the esophagus also may produce symptoms by inducing LM spasm. Using high-frequency intraluminal ultrasonography, Pehlivanov and colleagues[90] found that acid produced sustained esophageal contractions (SECs) marked by a significant increase in muscle thickness correlating with heartburn episodes. On esophageal manometry, there were no motor events associated with the SECs. Because manometry only measures circular muscle function, the investigators concluded that SECs were primarily a product of LM contraction.[90]

Sensitization also has a role in determining reflux perception. Acid sensitizes the esophagus in response to ensuing weakly acidic and nonacid reflux events.[85,89,91]

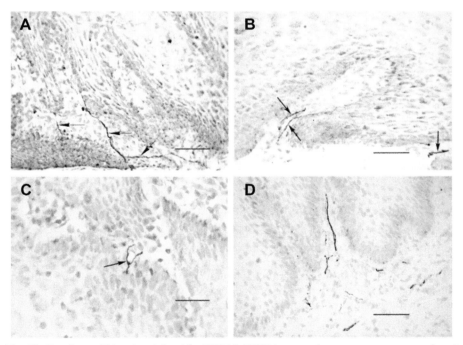

Fig. 12. Esophageal biopsies stained for TRPV-1. TRPV-1 expression appears more prominent in patients with EE (*A, B*) compared with normal controls (*C*). (*D*) Biopsy stained with peripherin confirms that TRPV-1 staining localizes to nerve fibers. Arrows demonstrate immunoreactive fibers in the papillae of areas with esophagitis. (*From* Matthews, P.J., et al., Increased capsaicin receptor TRPV1 nerve fibres in the inflamed human oesophagus. Eur J Gastroenterol Hepatol, 2004. 16(9): p. 897-902, with permission.)

Hu and colleagues[92] found that administration of acid in the duodenum decreased the pain threshold to esophageal electrical stimulation. Furthermore, duodenal infusion of fat decreases the chemosensitivity threshold to esophageal acid.[93] Pointing toward a central process, Schey and colleagues[94] found that sleep deprivation resulted in greater intensity and lower thresholds to pain response to esophageal acid.

SUMMARY

The pathophysiology of GERD starts with GER and culminates in a cascade of events. At the EGJ, compromise of the barrier formed by the CD and LES is the first step in GER. Once in the esophagus, the impact of reflux on epithelial defense depends on clearance mechanisms. Although degradation of the esophageal mucosa character-ized by DIS remains the prevailing mechanism, recent observations point to T lymphocyte–mediated inflammation. The process by which reflux interacts with sen-sory afferents remains to be elucidated. Further research will be required to under-stand how acid and central factors such as anxiety and sleep affect symptom perception.

REFERENCES

1. Hungin APS, Molloy-Bland M, Scarpignato C. Revisiting Montreal: new insights into symptoms and their causes, and implications for the future of GERD. Am J Gastroenterol 2019;114(3):414–21.
2. Mittal RK, Balaban DH, Epstein FH. The esophagogastric junction. N Engl J Med 1997;336:924–32.
3. Lerut T, Coosemans W, Decaluwe H, et al. The anatomy of the esophagus 2016. Available at: https://basicmedicalkey.com/the-anatomy-of-the-esophagus/. Ac-cessed August 29, 2019.
4. Stein HJ, Liebermann-Meffert D, DeMeester TR, et al. Three-dimensional pres-sure image and muscular structure of the human lower esophageal sphincter. Surgery 1995;117(6):692–8.
5. Mittal RK, Zifan A, Kumar D, et al. Functional morphology of the lower esophageal sphincter and crural diaphragm determined by three-dimensional high-resolution esophago-gastric junction pressure profile and CT imaging. Am J Physiol Gastro-intest Liver Physiol 2017;313(3):G212–9.
6. Mittal RK, Rochester DF, McCallum RW. Effect of the diaphragmatic contrac-tion on lower oesophageal sphincter pressure in man. Gut 1987;28(12):1564–8.
7. Eherer AJ, Netolitzky F, Högenauer C, et al. Positive effect of abdominal breathing exercise on gastroesophageal reflux disease: a randomized, controlled study. Am J Gastroenterol 2012;107(3):372–8.
8. Diamant NE. Pathophysiology of gastroesophageal reflux disease. GI Motility On-line 2006.
9. Cohen S, Harris LD. The lower esophageal sphincter. Gastroenterology 1972;63(6):1066–73.
10. Nicodeme F, Pipa-Muniz M, Khanna K, et al. Quantifying esophagogastric junc-tion contractility with a novel HRM topographic metric, the EGJ-Contractile Inte-gral: normative values and preliminary evaluation in PPI non-responders. Neurogastroenterol Motil 2014;26(3):353–60.
11. Jasper D, Freitas-Queiroz N, Hollenstein M, et al. Prolonged measurement im-proves the assessment of the barrier function of the esophago-gastric junction

by high-resolution manometry. Neurogastroenterol Motil 2017;29(2). https://doi.org/10.1111/nmo.12925.

12. Pandolfino JE, Curry J, Shi G, et al. Restoration of normal distensive characteristics of the esophagogastric junction after fundoplication. Ann Surg 2005; 242(1):43–8.

13. Tolone S, de Cassan C, de Bortoli N, et al. Esophagogastric junction morphology is associated with a positive impedance-pH monitoring in patients with GERD. Neurogastroenterol Motil 2015;27(8):1175–82.

14. Kahrilas PJ, Dodds WJ, Hogan WJ, et al. Esophageal peristaltic dysfunction in peptic esophagitis. Gastroenterology 1986;91(4):897–904.

15. Katzka DA, Sidhu M, Castell DO. Hypertensive lower esophageal sphincter pressures and gastroesophageal reflux: an apparent paradox that is not unusual. Am J Gastroenterol 1995;90(2):280–4.

16. Dent J, Holloway RH, Toouli J, et al. Mechanisms of lower oesophageal sphincter incompetence in patients with symptomatic gastrooesophageal reflux. Gut 1988; 29:1020–8.

17. Roman S, Holloway R, Keller J, et al. Validation of criteria for the definition of transient lower esophageal sphincter relaxations using high-resolution manometry. Neurogastroenterol Motil 2017;29(2). https://doi.org/10.1111/nmo.12920.

18. Pandolfino JE, Zhang QG, Ghosh SK, et al. Transient lower esophageal sphincter relaxations and reflux: mechanistic analysis using concurrent fluoroscopy and high-resolution manometry. Gastroenterology 2006;131(6):1725–33.

19. Dogan I, Bhargava V, Liu J, et al. Axial stretch: a novel mechanism of the lower esophageal sphincter relaxation. Am J Physiol Gastrointest Liver Physiol 2007; 292(1):G329–34.

20. Patel N, Jiang Y, Mittal RK, et al. Circular and longitudinal muscles shortening indicates sliding patterns during peristalsis and transient lower esophageal sphincter relaxation. Am J Physiol Gastrointest Liver Physiol 2015;309(5): G360–7.

21. Mittal RK, Fisher MJ. Electrical and mechanical inhibition of the crural diaphragm during transient relaxation of the lower esophageal sphincter. Gastroenterology 1990;99(5):1265–8.

22. Mittal RK, Stewart WR, Schirmer BD. Effect of a catheter in the pharynx on the frequency of transient lower esophageal sphincter relaxations. Gastroenterology 1992;103(4):1236–40.

23. Piche T, des Varannes SB, Sacher-Huvelin S, et al. Colonic fermentation influences lower esophageal sphincter function in gastroesophageal reflux disease. Gastroenterology 2003;124(4):894–902.

24. Zhang Q, Horowitz M, Rigda R, et al. Effect of hyperglycemia on triggering of transient lower esophageal sphincter relaxations. Am J Physiol Gastrointest Liver Physiol 2004;286(5):G797–803.

25. Kahrilas PJ, Gupta RR. Mechanisms of acid reflux associated with cigarette smoking. Gut 1990;31(1):4–10.

26. Holloway RH, Kocyan P, Dent J. Provocation of transient lower esophageal sphincter relaxations by meals in patients with symptomatic gastroesophageal reflux. Dig Dis Sci 1991;36(8):1034–9.

27. Herregods TV, Bredenoord AJ, Smout AJ. Pathophysiology of gastroesophageal reflux disease: new understanding in a new era. Neurogastroenterol Motil 2015; 27(9):1202–13.

28. Goyal RKM, Raj K. Sphincter mechanisms at the lower end of the esophagus. GI Motility Online 2006.

29. Scheffer RC, Akkermans LM, Bais JE, et al. Elicitation of transient lower oesopha-geal sphincter relaxations in response to gastric distension and meal ingestion. Neurogastroenterol Motil 2002;14(6):647–55.
30. Pauwels A, Altan E, Tack J. The gastric accommodation response to meal intake determines the occurrence of transient lower esophageal sphincter relaxations and reflux events in patients with gastro-esophageal reflux disease. Neurogas-troenterol Motil 2014;26(4):581–8.
31. Xiao YL, Peng S, Tao J, et al. Prevalence and symptom pattern of pathologic esophageal acid reflux in patients with functional dyspepsia based on the Rome III criteria. Am J Gastroenterol 2010;105(12):2626–31.
32. Camilleri M, Parkman HP, Shafi MA, et al. Clinical guideline: management of gas-troparesis. Am J Gastroenterol 2013;108(1):18–37 [quiz: 38].
33. Mittal RK, Holloway RH, Penagini R, et al. Transient lower esophageal sphincter relaxation. Gastroenterology 1995;109(2):601–10.
34. Scheffer RC, Wassenaar EB, Herwaarden MA, et al. Relationship between the mechanism of gastro-oesophageal reflux and oesophageal acid exposure in pa-tients with reflux disease. Neurogastroenterol Motil 2005;17(5):654–62.
35. Liu J, Pehlivanov N, Mittal RK. Baclofen blocks LES relaxation and crural dia-phragm inhibition by esophageal and gastric distension in cats. Am J Physiol Gastrointest Liver Physiol 2002;283(6):G1276–81.
36. Ireland AC, Holloway RH, Toouli J, et al. Mechanisms underlying the antireflux ac-tion of fundoplication. Gut 1993;34(3):303–8.
37. Jones MP, Sloan SS, Rabine JC, et al. Hiatal hernia size is the dominant determi-nant of esophagitis presence and severity in gastroesophageal reflux disease. Am J Gastroenterol 2001;96(6):1711–7.
38. van Herwaarden MA, Samsom M, Smout AJ. Excess gastroesophageal reflux in patients with hiatus hernia is caused by mechanisms other than transient LES re-laxations. Gastroenterology 2000;119(6):1439–46.
39. van Herwaarden MA, Samsom M, Smout AJ. The role of hiatus hernia in gastro-oesophageal reflux disease. Eur J Gastroenterol Hepatol 2004;16(9):831–5.
40. Gyawali CP, Roman S, Bredenoord AJ, et al. Classification of esophageal motor findings in gastro-esophageal reflux disease: conclusions from an international consensus group. Neurogastroenterol Motil 2017;29(12). https://doi.org/10.1111/nmo.13104.
41. Pandolfino JE, Kim H, Ghosh SK, et al. High-resolution manometry of the EGJ: an analysis of crural diaphragm function in GERD. Am J Gastroenterol 2007;102(5):1056–63.
42. Kahrilas PJ, Shi G, Manka M, et al. Increased frequency of transient lower esoph-ageal sphincter relaxation induced by gastric distention in reflux patients with hi-atal hernia. Gastroenterology 2000;118(4):688–95.
43. Pandolfino JE, Shi G, Trueworthy B, et al. Esophagogastric junction opening dur-ing relaxation distinguishes nonhernia reflux patients, hernia patients, and normal subjects. Gastroenterology 2003;125(4):1018–24.
44. Carlson DA. Functional lumen imaging probe: the FLIP side of esophageal dis-ease. Curr Opin Gastroenterol 2016;32(4):310–8.
45. Kwiatek MA, Pandolfino JE, Hirano I, et al. Esophagogastric junction distensibility assessed with an endoscopic functional luminal imaging probe (EndoFLIP). Gas-trointest Endosc 2010;72(2):272–8.
46. Boeckxstaens G. The relationship between the acid pocket and GERD. Gastroen-terol Hepatol (N Y) 2013;9(9):595–6.

47. Fletcher J, Wirz A, Young J, et al. Unbuffered highly acidic gastric juice exists at the gastroesophageal junction after a meal. Gastroenterology 2001;121(4): 775–83.
48. Pandolfino JE, Zhang Q, Ghosh SK, et al. Acidity surrounding the squamocolumnar junction in GERD patients: "acid pocket" versus "acid film". Am J Gastroenterol 2007;102(12):2633–41.
49. Clarke AT, Wirz AA, Manning JJ, et al. Severe reflux disease is associated with an enlarged unbuffered proximal gastric acid pocket. Gut 2008;57(3):292–7.
50. Beaumont H, Bennink RJ, de Jong J, et al. The position of the acid pocket as a major risk factor for acidic reflux in healthy subjects and patients with GORD. Gut 2010;59(4):441–51.
51. Rohof WO, Bennink RJ, Boeckxstaens GE. Proton pump inhibitors reduce the size and acidity of the acid pocket in the stomach. Clin Gastroenterol Hepatol 2014;12(7):1101–7.e1.
52. Scarpellini E, Boecxstaens V, Farré R, et al. Effect of baclofen on the acid pocket at the gastroesophageal junction. Dis Esophagus 2015;28(5):488–95.
53. De Ruigh A, Roman S, Chen J, et al. Gaviscon Double Action Liquid (antacid & alginate) is more effective than antacid in controlling post-prandial oesophageal acid exposure in GERD patients: a double-blind crossover study. Aliment Pharmacol Ther 2014;40(5):531–7.
54. Sweis R, Kaufman E, Anggiansah A, et al. Post-prandial reflux suppression by a raft-forming alginate (Gaviscon Advance) compared to a simple antacid documented by magnetic resonance imaging and pH-impedance monitoring: mechanistic assessment in healthy volunteers and randomised, controlled, double-blind study in reflux patients. Aliment Pharmacol Ther 2013;37(11): 1093–102.
55. Thomas E, Wade A, Crawford G, et al. Randomised clinical trial: relief of upper gastrointestinal symptoms by an acid pocket-targeting alginate-antacid (Gaviscon Double Action) - a double-blind, placebo-controlled, pilot study in gastro-oesophageal reflux disease. Aliment Pharmacol Ther 2014;39(6):595–602.
56. Sloan S, Kahrilas PJ. Impairment of esophageal emptying with hiatal hernia. Gastroenterology 1991;100(3):596–605.
57. Bredenoord AJ, Pandolfino JE, Smout AJ. Gastro-oesophageal reflux disease. Lancet 2013;381(9881):1933–42.
58. Curcic J, Roy S, Schwizer A, et al. Abnormal structure and function of the esophagogastric junction and proximal stomach in gastroesophageal reflux disease. Am J Gastroenterol 2014;109(5):658–67.
59. Barlow WJ, Orlando RC. The pathogenesis of heartburn in nonerosive reflux disease: a unifying hypothesis. Gastroenterology 2005;128(3):771–8.
60. Frierson HF Jr. Histology in the diagnosis of reflux esophagitis. Gastroenterol Clin North Am 1990;19(3):631–44.
61. Woodland P, Sifrim D. Esophageal mucosal integrity in nonerosive reflux disease. J Clin Gastroenterol 2014;48(1):6–12.
62. Jovov B, Que J, Tobey NA, et al. Role of E-cadherin in the pathogenesis of gastroesophageal reflux disease. Am J Gastroenterol 2011;106(6):1039–47.
63. Tobey NA, Gambling TM, Vanegas XC, et al. Physicochemical basis for dilated intercellular spaces in non-erosive acid-damaged rabbit esophageal epithelium. Dis Esophagus 2008;21(8):757–64.
64. van Malenstein H, Farre R, Sifrim D. Esophageal dilated intercellular spaces (DIS) and nonerosive reflux disease. Am J Gastroenterol 2008;103(4):1021–8.

65. Kessing BF, Bredenoord AJ, Weijenborg PW, et al. Esophageal acid exposure decreases intraluminal baseline impedance levels. Am J Gastroenterol 2011; 106(12):2093–7.

66. Xie C, Sifrim D, Li Y, et al. Esophageal baseline impedance reflects mucosal integrity and predicts symptomatic outcome with proton pump inhibitor treatment. J Neurogastroenterol Motil 2018;24(1):43–50.

67. Kandulski A, Weigt J, Caro C, et al. Esophageal intraluminal baseline impedance differentiates gastroesophageal reflux disease from functional heartburn. Clin Gastroenterol Hepatol 2015;13(6):1075–81.

68. Souza RF, Huo X, Mittal V, et al. Gastroesophageal reflux might cause esophagitis through a cytokine-mediated mechanism rather than caustic acid injury. Gastroenterology 2009;137(5):1776–84.

69. Dunbar KB, Agoston AT, Odze RD, et al. Association of acute gastroesophageal reflux disease with esophageal histologic changes. JAMA 2016;315(19): 2104–12.

70. Huo X, Agoston AT, Dunbar KB, et al. Hypoxia-inducible factor-2alpha plays a role in mediating oesophagitis in GORD. Gut 2017;66(9):1542–54.

71. Singh P, Taylor RH, Colin-Jones DG. Esophageal motor dysfunction and acid exposure in reflux esophagitis are more severe if Barrett's metaplasia is present. Am J Gastroenterol 1994;89(3):349–56.

72. Timmer R, Breumelhof R, Nadorp JH, et al. Esophageal motility in low-grade reflux esophagitis, evaluated by stationary and 24-hour ambulatory manometry. Am J Gastroenterol 1993;88(6):837–41.

73. Savarino E, Gemignani L, Pohl D, et al. Oesophageal motility and bolus transit abnormalities increase in parallel with the severity of gastro-oesophageal reflux disease. Aliment Pharmacol Ther 2011;34(4):476–86.

74. Helm JF, Dodds WJ, Pelc LR, et al. Effect of esophageal emptying and saliva on clearance of acid from the esophagus. N Engl J Med 1984;310(5):284–8.

75. Frazzoni M, Manta R, Mirante VG, et al. Esophageal chemical clearance is impaired in gastro-esophageal reflux disease–a 24-h impedance-pH monitoring assessment. Neurogastroenterol Motil 2013;25(5):399–406, e295.

76. Frazzoni M, Savarino E, de Bortoli N, et al. Analyses of the post-reflux swallow-induced peristaltic wave index and nocturnal baseline impedance parameters increase the diagnostic yield of patients with reflux disease. Clin Gastroenterol Hepatol 2016;14(1):40–6.

77. Schoeman MN, Holloway RH. Integrity and characteristics of secondary oesophageal peristalsis in patients with gastro-oesophageal reflux disease. Gut 1995;36(4):499–504.

78. Carlson DA, Kathpalia P, Craft J, et al. The relationship between esophageal acid exposure and the esophageal response to volumetric distention. Neurogastroenterol Motil 2018;30(3). https://doi.org/10.1111/nmo.13240.

79. Caterina MJ, Schumacher MA, Tominaga M, et al. The capsaicin receptor: a heat-activated ion channel in the pain pathway. Nature 1997;389(6653):816–24.

80. Szallasi A, Blumberg PM. Vanilloid (Capsaicin) receptors and mechanisms. Pharmacol Rev 1999;51(2):159–212.

81. Geppetti P, Trevisani M. Activation and sensitisation of the vanilloid receptor: role in gastrointestinal inflammation and function. Br J Pharmacol 2004;141(8): 1313–20.

82. Bhat YM, Bielefeldt K. Capsaicin receptor (TRPV1) and non-erosive reflux disease. Eur J Gastroenterol Hepatol 2006;18(3):263–70.

83. Matthews PJ, Aziz Q, Facer P, et al. Increased capsaicin receptor TRPV1 nerve fibres in the inflamed human oesophagus. Eur J Gastroenterol Hepatol 2004; 16(9):897–902.

84. Lee RH, Korsapati H, Bhalla V, et al. Esophageal submucosal injection of capsaicin but not acid induces symptoms in normal subjects. J Neurogastroenterol Motil 2016;22(3):436–43.

85. Bredenoord AJ, Weusten BL, Curvers WL, et al. Determinants of perception of heartburn and regurgitation. Gut 2006;55(3):313–8.

86. Bredenoord AJ, Weusten BL, Timmer R, et al. Characteristics of gastroesophageal reflux in symptomatic patients with and without excessive esophageal acid exposure. Am J Gastroenterol 2006;101(11):2470–5.

87. Cicala M, Emerenziani S, Caviglia R, et al. Intra-oesophageal distribution and perception of acid reflux in patients with non-erosive gastro-oesophageal reflux disease. Aliment Pharmacol Ther 2003;18(6):605–13.

88. Emerenziani S, Ribolsi M, Sifrim D, et al. Regional oesophageal sensitivity to acid and weakly acidic reflux in patients with non-erosive reflux disease. Neurogastroenterol Motil 2009;21(3):253–8.

89. Zerbib F, Duriez A, Roman S, et al. Determinants of gastro-oesophageal reflux perception in patients with persistent symptoms despite proton pump inhibitors. Gut 2008;57(2):156–60.

90. Pehlivanov N, Liu J, Mittal RK. Sustained esophageal contraction: a motor correlate of heartburn symptom. Am J Physiol Gastrointest Liver Physiol 2001;281(3): G743–51.

91. Emerenziani S, Ribolsi M, Guarino MP, et al. Acid reflux episodes sensitize the esophagus to perception of weakly acidic and mixed reflux in non-erosive reflux disease patients. Neurogastroenterol Motil 2014;26(1):108–14.

92. Hu WH, Martin CJ, Talley NJ. Intraesophageal acid perfusion sensitizes the esophagus to mechanical distension: a Barostat study. Am J Gastroenterol 2000;95(9):2189–94.

93. Meyer JH, Lembo A, Elashoff JD, et al. Duodenal fat intensifies the perception of heartburn. Gut 2001;49(5):624–8.

94. Schey R, Dickman R, Parthasarathy S, et al. Sleep deprivation is hyperalgesic in patients with gastroesophageal reflux disease. Gastroenterology 2007;133(6): 1787–95.

Personalized Approach in the Work-up and Management of Gastroesophageal Reflux Disease

Rena Yadlapati, MD, MSHS[a],*, John E. Pandolfino, MD, MSCI[b]

KEYWORDS

- Reflux • Proton pump inhibitor • Esophageal manometry • Esophagitis
- Hiatal hernia • Functional heartburn • Supragastric belching
- Transient lower esophageal sphincter relaxation

KEY POINTS

- Gastroesophageal reflux disease (GERD) is a prevalent disorder associated with serious quality-of-life impairment and health care expenditure.
- Patients with GERD present with heterogeneous phenotypes and require personalized diagnostic and treatment strategies.
- A stepwise framework to phenotype GERD is intended to optimize phenotypic yield and minimize risk and cost.
  - Step 1 is to characterize symptom profile and response to proton pump inhibitor therapy.
  - Step 2 is indicated when symptom response is inadequate, patient presentation is atypical, and/or warning signs/symptoms are present. Step 2 is endoscopic evaluation for mucosal and anatomic integrity, and to assess for alternative diagnoses.
  - Step 3 is indicated in the absence of erosive reflux disease or severe disruption of the antireflux barrier. Step 3 is ambulatory reflux monitoring, typically off acid suppression, to characterize reflux burden and evaluate for reflux hypersensitivity.
  - Step 4 is indicated if the GERD phenotype remains unclear. Step 4 is esophageal function testing with high-resolution impedance manometry with or without pH impedance testing to assess for reflux mechanism, peristaltic clearance, and alternate sources of symptoms.

Author Contributions: Drs R. Yadlapati and J.E. Pandolfino performed a literature review and data analysis, drafted the initial article, made meaningful revisions, and approved the final version of the article.

Research Support: Dr R. Yadlapati is supported by the ACG Research Institute – Junior Faculty Development Award (R. Yadlapati). Dr R. Yadlapati and Dr J.E. Pandolfino are supported by the NIH R01DK092217-04A1 (J.E. Pandolfino).

[a] Division of Gastroenterology, University of California San Diego, 9500 Gilman Drive MC 0956, La Jolla, CA 92093, USA; [b] Division of Gastroenterology and Hepatology, Northwestern University Feinberg School of Medicine, 676 North St. Clair Street, Chicago, IL 60611, USA
* Corresponding author.
E-mail address: ryadlapati@ucsd.edu

Gastrointest Endoscopy Clin N Am 30 (2020) 227–238
https://doi.org/10.1016/j.giec.2019.12.002

giendo.theclinics.com

INTRODUCTION

Gastroesophageal reflux disease (GERD) affects 1 in 5 Americans and is one of the most common diagnoses managed in the outpatient gastroenterology clinic.[1,2] According to the Montreal Consensus, GERD is defined as the presence of troublesome symptoms and/or complications that develop because of retrograde reflux of gastric contents in the esophagus.[2] Historically, GERD management has relied on empiric treatment approaches, and proved unsuccessful. Traditionally, GERD is diagnosed based on presence of symptoms and managed reflexively with acid-suppressive medication, particularly proton pump inhibitors (PPIs). However, up to 40% of patients treated with PPIs may have incomplete or no symptom response to therapy.[3] Because various symptoms (eg, heartburn, regurgitation, chest pain, globus, dysphagia, throat symptoms, cough, belching) can be attributed to GERD, and a multitude of mechanisms can result in gastroesophageal reflux physiology, individuals with GERD respond differently to a single-pronged treatment approach.

Recent advancements in esophageal physiology and psychology have led to the development of sophisticated diagnostic tools to evaluate GERD. Clinical sites across the world have adopted these diagnostic tools, such as pH monitoring and high-resolution manometry systems, to evaluate esophageal disorders. At the same time, therapeutic options for GERD beyond PPI therapy and laparoscopic fundoplication have expanded. Treatment options for GERD now span behavioral interventions, various pharmacologic applications, and minimally invasive endoluminal and laparoscopic techniques. These state-of-the-art concepts, diagnostic tools, and treatment options offer tremendous opportunity for personalizing the management of GERD. Therefore, this article reviews a personalized approach for the evaluation and management of GERD.

THEORY OF PERSONALIZATION IN GASTROESOPHAGEAL REFLUX DISEASE

Patients with GERD symptoms can be classified based on multiple factors, including clinical history (predominant symptom and response to PPI), endoscopic findings (gastroesophageal flap valve, hiatal hernia, esophagitis), ambulatory reflux testing (acid exposure, reflux events), and esophageal function (reflux clearance, alternate causes of symptoms). Different permutations of these factors can yield more than 50 classifications, or phenotypes, of GERD. This concept is akin to a game of poker in which a particular combination of cards (factors) may lead to different hands of cards (phenotypes of GERD) (**Fig. 1**). In poker, betting uses probability theory to ascertain the odds of the particular poker hand. Similarly, in a phenotype approach to personalizing the management of GERD, the treatment decision is based on the predicted outcome for the particular phenotype of GERD.

FOUR STEPS OF PHENOTYPING IN A PERSONALIZED APPROACH FOR GASTROESOPHAGEAL REFLUX DISEASE

The proposed personalized approach for GERD uses a stepwise method that optimizes phenotypic yield and outcome, and minimizes invasiveness, risk, and cost (**Fig. 2**). Continuing with the poker analogy, in Texas hold'em, cards are revealed to players in a stepwise method, and bets are placed at each step. At any step a player may decide to go all in (bet everything) given very high odds of winning, or alternatively fold given very high odds of losing. Similarly, throughout the stepwise method for phenotyping GERD, clinicians may at any point elect to halt further testing (akin to folding or going all in) and proceed with management if the information available identifies a distinct GERD phenotype.

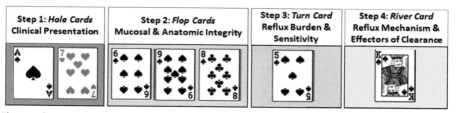

Fig. 1. The combination of factors in phenotyping GERD are akin to the combination of cards in a game of poker. Phenotypes of GERD, or a combination of cards, are revealed in a stepwise fashion. At any step, a provider, or player, may decide to stop further evaluation and treat given the very high odds of outcome for a certain phenotype.

Step 1: Clinical Presentation to Assess Symptom and Response to Proton Pump Inhibitor (Hole Cards)

A good history is crucial in step 1 of the evaluation of GERD. This history is typically focused on the symptom presentation, the response to a PPI trial, and also other key factors that may implicate and modulate reflux severity, such as obesity and underlying comorbidities such as scleroderma or sleep apnea. In addition, an underlying assessment of visceral anxiety and hypervigilance may be important clues in developing the phenotypes and treatment strategies because these factors will modulate response across all GERD phenotypes. Typically, GERD is initially diagnosed based on symptom presentation and further classified based on response to antireflux treatment. Clinically diagnosed symptomatic syndromes of GERD include typical reflux syndromes in the setting of heartburn and/or regurgitation, or reflux chest pain syndrome.[2] Further, clinically diagnosed GERD may be caused by extraesophageal syndromes such as reflux cough, reflux laryngitis, or reflux asthma[2] (**Fig. 3**). The therapeutic gain of PPI therapy, the mainstay treatment of clinically suspected GERD, compared with placebo in treating GERD syndromes varies.[3,4] When esophagitis is not present, therapeutic efficacy is greatest for heartburn symptoms, less so for regurgitation or chest pain, and least for

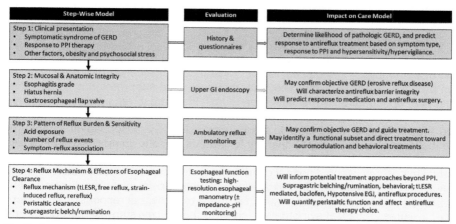

Fig. 2. Four steps of phenotyping in GERD to define important biomarkers and clinical predictors of treatment and disease outcomes. GI, gastrointestinal; tLESR, transient lower esophageal sphincter relaxation.

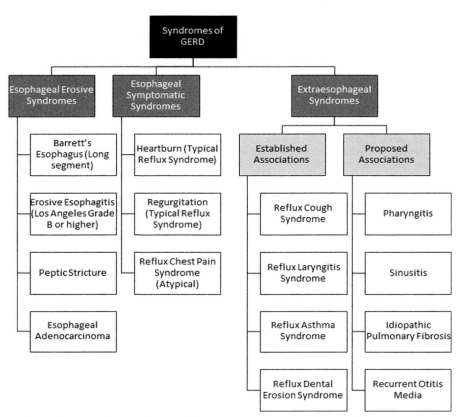

Fig. 3. Syndromes of GERD (adapted from the Montreal Classification) classify GERD as an esophageal syndrome or extraesophageal syndrome. Esophageal syndromes may be those associated with esophageal injury or based on symptom presentation. (*From* Vakil N, van Zanten SV, Kahrilas P, et al. The Montreal definition and classification of gastroesophageal reflux disease: a global evidence-based consensus. Am J Gastroenterol 2006;101:1900-20; with permission.)

extraesophageal syndromes.[5] Variation in outcomes of PPI therapy is likely a function of pathophysiologic mechanism. For instance, acidification of the esophagus can provoke heartburn symptoms, and, therefore, acid suppression is an effective treatment option for acid-mediated heartburn.[6] In contrast, regurgitation is a function of gastroesophageal reflux volume rather than the acidic nature of refluxate, and thus it is less responsive to acid suppression. Extraesophageal symptoms are the least responsive to PPI therapy for various reasons. In up to 60% of cases, extraesophageal symptoms are caused by nonreflux conditions such as environmental exposures, sinopulmonary conditions, and voice use.[7] Studies also suggest that higher pH levels can impart noxious stimuli and injury in the hypopharynx compared with the distal esophagus.[8] For these reasons, the response to PPI therapy for extraesophageal symptoms is close to that of placebo.[9,10] Therefore, clinical assessment of esophageal and/or extraesophageal symptoms, and response to PPI therapy, is an important initial component in GERD phenotyping. This component is combined with the underlying patient characteristics that may be related to the development of heartburn, such as recent weight gain and new medications that reduce lower esophageal sphincter (LES) pressure.

Step 2: Upper Gastrointestinal Endoscopy to Assess Mucosal and Anatomic Integrity (Flop Cards)

Information from step 1 helps to guide the need for upper gastrointestinal (GI) endoscopy (step 2). Upper GI endoscopy is the next step for patients with typical reflux symptoms without adequate response to PPI therapy, atypical reflux symptoms, as well as warning signs or symptoms such as dysphagia, GI bleeding, weight loss, or iron deficiency anemia.[11] First, endoscopic assessment of the esophagus determines presence and severity of erosive reflux disease. The presence of Los Angeles (LA) C or D esophagitis, long-segment Barrett's esophagus, and/or peptic stricture provides objective confirmation of pathologic GERD and signifies a higher likelihood of response to antireflux therapy.[12] Although the Lyon Consensus considers LA B inconclusive for GERD, the finding of LA B esophagitis along with typical symptoms has a high likelihood of underlying reflux unless alternative factors are noted, such as eosinophilic esophagitis, or a dermatologic or nonpeptic esophagitis pattern.

Next, endoscopic assessment of the integrity of the antireflux barrier affects the likelihood for medical management to succeed. The antireflux barrier is a high-pressure zone comprising the LES attached to the crural diaphragm via the phrenoesophageal ligament, which forms a tight gastroesophageal flap valve to prevent pathologic gastroesophageal reflux.[13] Disruption to the antireflux barrier may lead to increased reflux burden and acid exposure. Axial separation between the crural diaphragm and LES results in a hiatal hernia. Hiatal hernia, as well as reduced tonicity of the intrinsic LES, reduces the integrity of the gastroesophageal flap valve mechanism. Therefore, endoscopic assessment of the antireflux barrier via characterization of hernia, if present; measurement of length of separation between the diaphragmatic pinch (crural diaphragm) and the proximal extent of the gastric folds (LES); and grading of the gastroesophageal flap valve are important steps in phenotyping GERD.[13]

Endoscopy also enables evaluation of alternate sources of esophageal symptoms, such as eosinophilic esophagitis, mechanical obstruction, other nonpeptic esophagitis, or peptic ulcer disease.

Step 3: Reflux Monitoring to Characterize Pattern of Reflux Burden and Reflux Sensitivity (Turn Card)

When erosive reflux disease is not present, the next step is to characterize the reflux burden with reflux monitoring to assess for acid exposure, reflux events, and association between symptom perception and reflux events.[14] Ambulatory reflux monitoring is available as 24-hour transnasal catheter recording with or without impedance monitoring, and wireless pH monitoring with prolonged monitoring capabilities. When the pretest likelihood of GERD is low, defined by the Lyon Consensus as lack of erosive reflux disease, ambulatory reflux monitoring is performed off acid suppression in order to establish presence of GERD at baseline.[15] In contrast, if the pretest likelihood of GERD is high, defined by objective evidence of reflux by way of erosive reflux disease on endoscopy or previous positive reflux monitoring, ambulatory reflux monitoring is performed on acid suppression to evaluate for refractory GERD (**Fig. 4**).[16]

According to the recent Lyon Consensus for GERD, esophageal acid exposure time greater than 6.0% is consistent with acidic gastroesophageal reflux disease, acid

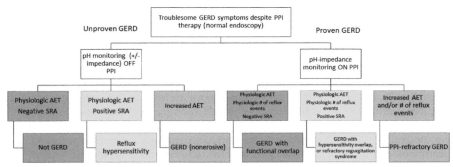

Fig. 4. Reflux monitoring for PPI nonresponse for patients with nonerosive GERD symptoms. For patients with unproven GERD, ambulatory reflux monitoring off PPI is recommended to assess for presence or absence of pathologic acid exposure time (AET) and symptom-reflux association (SRA) in order to phenotype GERD. In setting of previously proven GERD, ambulatory reflux monitoring with pH impedance on PPI is recommended to identify whether GERD with a functional or hypersensitivity overlap is present, whether a regurgitation syndrome is present, or whether PPI-refractory GERD is present.

exposure time less than 4.0% is physiologic, and acid exposure times between 4.0% and 6.0% are inconclusive and require further testing. Also, per the Lyon Consensus, more than 80 reflux events is consistent with increased reflux burden, less than 40 reflux events is physiologic, and between 40 and 80 is inconclusive.[16] These values are levels of confidence, or the amount of money you would wager, that the patient has underlying GERD.

Furthermore, reflux monitoring evaluates the association between reflux events and symptom perception. A positive symptom index (SI) (50% or more of a symptom is associated with a reflux event) and a positive symptom association probability (SAP) (>95%) are consistent with positive symptom-reflux association. When acid exposure and reflux events are within normal limits, a symptom-reflux association indicates esophageal hypersensitivity.[16]

Esophageal hypersensitivity is symptom perception of heartburn/chest pain under nonpathologic reflux settings, and is a function of allodynia and hyperalgesia caused by central and peripheral sensitization. As such, treatments to modulate neural perception, such as behavioral interventions or low-dose antidepressants, are therapies for esophageal hypersensitivity.[6] In contrast, patients with a positive symptom association for the perception of regurgitation on PPI therapy may have significant nonacid reflux burden and this is different than reflux hypersensitivity because it is most commonly caused by overt defects in the antireflux barrier.

Therefore, for patients with unproven GERD, reflux monitoring can classify reflux burden as nonerosive reflux disease with acid burden, reflux hypersensitivity, regurgitation of acid or nonacid refluxate, or absence of GERD.

Step 4: Esophageal Function Testing to Identify Reflux Mechanism, Characterize Peristaltic Clearance, and Evaluate for Alternate Causes (River Card)

Esophageal function testing with esophageal manometry with or without impedance-pH monitoring can provide adjunctive qualitative assessments in GERD. Esophageal manometry is another method to evaluate the antireflux barrier, and to additionally characterize the gastroesophageal reflux mechanism. For instance, esophageal manometry can identify transient LES relaxations (tLESRs), prolonged relaxations in the LES associated with inhibition of the crural diaphragm that occur in response to gastric distention in the absence of a swallow.[17,18] tLESRs are the primary mechanism of initiating reflux in the context of an intact antireflux barrier, and can be pharmacologically inhibited with GABA agonists.[18–21] When the antireflux barrier is disrupted, esophageal manometry may identify pathologic reflux as a function of strain-induced reflux, free reflux, or rereflux of contents from a nonreducible hiatal hernia.[22] In these cases, pharmacologic treatment options are limited and may indicate the need for mechanical restoration of the crural diaphragm.

Manometric properties can also be assessed following a meal to evaluate for behavioral conditions such as rumination or supragastric belching.[23,24] The sensitivity and specificity of high-resolution impedance manometry for diagnosis of rumination are 80% and 100%, and when the pretest suspicion for rumination is high, postprandial testing on manometry can identify rumination in up to 20% of cases.[17,25,26] Supragastric belching is identifiable on pH impedance monitoring and high-resolution impedance manometry.[27]

Further, esophageal manometry provides valuable assessment of peristaltic function and esophageal clearance properties, and helps to predict response to treatment and risk of posttreatment symptoms. For instance, a reduced distal contractile integral (<450 mm Hg-s-cm) in most swallows indicates a hypomotile esophageal motor condition, and an insufficient distal contractile integral following multiple rapid swallows indicates reduced peristaltic reserve.[28,29] Hypomotile patterns have an increased risk of postfundoplication dysphagia, and in these cases tailored fundoplication techniques or alternative antireflux procedures should be considered.

THERAPEUTIC STRATEGIES PERSONALIZED TO GASTROESOPHAGEAL REFLUX DISEASE PHENOTYPE

GERD is not one and the same, and, as such, all treatments available to manage GERD are not appropriate across all patients. Therapeutic strategies should be personalized to the GERD phenotype. Examples of different scenarios of patients with GERD are discussed here. Through a stepwise phenotype approach, a personalized therapeutic strategy for the distinct GERD phenotype is established. Other articles in this issue describe in detail therapeutic options for GERD, such as acid suppression, endoluminal interventions, and surgery.

Example 1 (**Fig. 5**A): a 65-year-old man is referred to clinic for:

1. Heartburn and regurgitation that responds partially to PPI therapy (hole cards).
2. He undergoes upper GI endoscopy, which reveals a 5-cm nonreducible hiatal hernia with grade IV gastroesophageal flap valve and LA D esophagitis (flop cards).
   - Thus, this patient's phenotype is typical reflux symptoms with partial PPI response, erosive reflux disease, and a severely disrupted antireflux barrier. At this point further diagnostic evaluation with reflux monitoring or esophageal function testing is not needed. The clinician can go all in without the turn or river card. Management should focus on optimizing acid suppression and mechanical restoration of the gastroesophageal flap valve.

Example 2 (**Fig. 5**B): a 65-year-old man is referred to clinic for:

1. Heartburn without response to PPI therapy and recent weight gain (hole cards).
2. He undergoes upper GI endoscopy, which reveals normal esophageal mucosa, a 0.5-cm sliding hiatal hernia, and grade II gastroesophageal flap valve (flop cards).

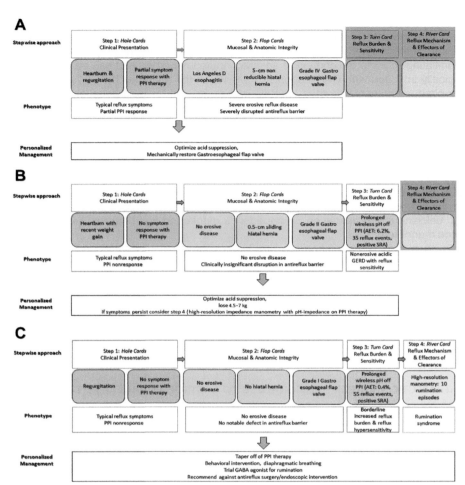

Fig. 5. Stepwise phenotype approach for 3 patient examples (A–C). (A) A 65-year-old man is referred for heartburn and regurgitation partially responsive to PPI (hole cards) and undergoes upper GI endoscopy, which reveals a 5-cm nonreducible hiatal hernia with grade IV gastroesophageal flap valve and LAD esophagitis (flop cards). This patient's phenotype is clear at this point (typical reflux symptoms with partial PPI response, erosive reflux disease, and a severely disrupted antireflux barrier), and thus phenotype-guided management can proceed without further evaluation. Management in this case hinges on optimizing acid suppression and mechanical restoration of the gastroesophageal flap valve. (B) A 65-year-old man with recent weight gain, heartburn, and no response to PPI therapy (hole cards) undergoes upper GI endoscopy, which reveals normal esophageal mucosa, a 0.5-cm sliding hiatal hernia, and grade II gastroesophageal flap valve (flop cards). The GERD phenotype is not clear at this point, and the next step is ambulatory reflux monitoring. Because the patient has a low pretest probability of GERD, the patient undergoes prolonged wireless pH monitoring off PPI therapy. The AET is increased. Thus, this patient's phenotype is heartburn symptoms with recent weight gain, PPI nonresponder with nonerosive acidic reflux disease. At this point management can be attempted without further diagnostic evaluation focused on weight loss and optimizing acid suppression. However, if symptoms persist, further evaluation with esophageal manometry and impedance-pH monitoring on PPI (river card) would be warranted. (C) A 65-year-old man is referred to clinic for regurgitation and no

3. The next step is ambulatory reflux monitoring. Because the patient has a low pre-test probability of GERD, the patient undergoes prolonged wireless pH monitoring off PPI therapy. The acid exposure is 6.2%, 35 reflux events per day, and there is a positive symptom-reflux association (SI, 75% and SAP, 98%) for 25 symptoms of heartburn.

- Thus, this patient's phenotype is heartburn symptoms with recent weight gain, PPI nonresponder with nonerosive reflux , likely acid predominant with component of reflux sensitivity. At this point management can be attempted without further diagnostic evaluation (bet high without river card), focused on weight loss and optimizing acid suppression. However, if the wager is whether or not to proceed with antireflux surgery, obtaining high-resolution manometry (river card) at this point is extremely important because this may help guide decisions on the type of antireflux intervention used to treat the underlying GERD. Because the patient's symptoms persist, the patient undergoes esophageal manometry and impedance-pH monitoring on PPI (river card). In this case, testing reveals frequent tLESRs with gastroesophageal reflux events, and controlled acid exposure on PPI. Adjunctive management in this case could include the addition of tLESR inhibition.

Example 3 (**Fig. 5C**): a 65-year-old man is referred to clinic for:

1. Regurgitation and no response to PPI therapy (hole cards).
2. He undergoes upper GI endoscopy, which reveals normal esophageal mucosa, no hiatal hernia, and grade I gastroesophageal flap valve (flop cards).
3. The next step is ambulatory reflux monitoring, which shows 55 reflux events, normal acid exposure, and positive symptom-reflux association for regurgitation (SI, 100%; SAP, 99%) (turn card).
   - Thus, the phenotype at this point is PPI nonresponder with regurgitation and borderline increased reflux burden. A mucosal protective agent can be added, but because you suspect rumination, and given borderline testing, you pursue additional testing.
4. High-resolution esophageal manometry and impedance-pH monitoring on PPI are performed and reveal 10 rumination episodes during the 60-minute postprandial testing period (river card).
   - Thus this patient is a PPI nonresponder with rumination, and management focuses on behavioral intervention, diaphragmatic breathing, and trial of GABA agonist.[30] In this case, the clinician refrains from referring for antireflux surgery.

---

response to PPI therapy (hole cards) and undergoes upper GI endoscopy, which reveals normal esophageal mucosa, no hiatal hernia, and grade I gastroesophageal flap valve (flop cards). The GERD phenotype is unclear and so the next step is ambulatory reflux monitoring, which shows an inconclusive number of reflux events, normal acid exposure, and positive SRA for regurgitation (SI, 100%; SAP, 99%) (turn card). Given inconclusive findings and suspicion for rumination, the next step is esophageal physiologic testing with manometry and pH impedance on PPI therapy, which uncovers rumination syndrome. At this point, the phenotype is clear (PPI nonresponder with rumination) and management focuses on behavioral intervention, diaphragmatic breathing, and trial of GABA agonist. In this case the clinician refrains from referring for antireflux surgery.

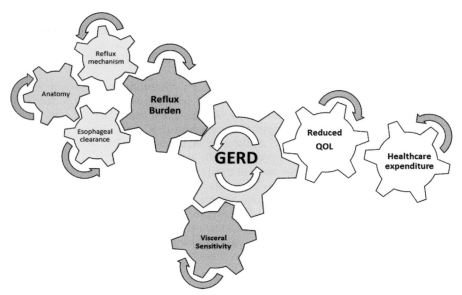

Fig. 6. Conceptual model of the interaction of the components of phenotyping in GERD that lead to reduced quality of life (QOL) and increased health care use.

SUMMARY

In summary, GERD is prevalent disorder and patients present with heterogeneous phenotypes that require personalized treatment strategies. Personalization of treatment of GERD requires an understanding of the patient's GERD phenotype. The framework to phenotype GERD hinges on a stepwise bayesian evaluation method that minimizes risk and cost, and maximizes phenotypic yield (see **Fig. 2**). The stepwise evaluation begins with characterization of symptom profile and response to PPI therapy. In cases of inadequate symptom response, the next step is endoscopic evaluation of mucosal and anatomic integrity. In the absence of erosive reflux disease and a severe disruption, the third step is ambulatory reflux monitoring, off PPI therapy in the case of unproven GERD, to characterize reflux burden and evaluate for esophageal hypersensitivity. At this juncture, if the GERD phenotype remains unclear, the next step is to perform esophageal function testing with high-resolution impedance manometry with or without pH impedance testing to evaluate for mechanism of gastroesophageal reflux event, peristaltic clearance from esophagus, and alternate sources of symptoms. Esophageal function testing is also a part of the preoperative evaluation for antireflux surgery. Therapeutic strategies should be focused on the GERD phenotype and begin with the least invasive and safest treatment options. In addition, factors focused on visceral anxiety and hypervigilance need to be addressed because these features can affect symptom severity and health care use. These treat-to-mechanism phenotype approaches to GERD are critical for reducing the serious health care burden of GERD that is generated from a combination of these important anatomic, physiologic, and psychological biomarkers (**Fig. 6**).

DISCLOSURE

Dr J.E. Pandolfino is a consultant for Crospon, Ironwood, Torax, Astra Zeneca, Takeda, Impleo, Medtronic, and Diversatek.

REFERENCES

1. Peery AF, Crockett SD, Barritt AS, et al. Burden of gastrointestinal, liver, and pancreatic diseases in the United States. Gastroenterology 2015;149: 1731–1741 e3.
2. Vakil N, van Zanten SV, Kahrilas P, et al. The Montreal definition and classification of gastroesophageal reflux disease: a global evidence-based consensus. Am J Gastroenterol 2006;101:1900–20 [quiz: 1943].
3. Bytzer P, Jones R, Vakil N, et al. Limited ability of the proton-pump inhibitor test to identify patients with gastroesophageal reflux disease. Clin Gastroenterol Hepatol 2012;10:1360–6.
4. de Bortoli N, Martinucci I, Savarino E, et al. Proton pump inhibitor responders who are not confirmed as GERD patients with impedance and pH monitoring: who are they? Neurogastroenterol Motil 2014;26:28–35.
5. Kahrilas PJ, Boeckxstaens G. Failure of reflux inhibitors in clinical trials: bad drugs or wrong patients? Gut 2012;61:1501–9.
6. Aziz Q, Fass R, Gyawali CP, et al. Functional esophageal disorders. Gastroenterology 2016 [pii:S0016-5085(16)00178-5].
7. de Bortoli N, Nacci A, Savarino E, et al. How many cases of laryngopharyngeal reflux suspected by laryngoscopy are gastroesophageal reflux disease-related? World J Gastroenterol 2012;18:4363–70.
8. Ang D, Ang TL, Teo EK, et al. Is impedance pH monitoring superior to the conventional 24-h pH meter in the evaluation of patients with laryngorespiratory symptoms suspected to be due to gastroesophageal reflux disease? J Dig Dis 2011;12:341–8.
9. Lechien JR, Saussez S, Schindler A, et al. Clinical outcomes of laryngopharyngeal reflux treatment: a systematic review and meta-analysis. Laryngoscope 2019; 129:1174–87.
10. Liu C, Wang H, Liu K. Meta-analysis of the efficacy of proton pump inhibitors for the symptoms of laryngopharyngeal reflux. Braz J Med Biol Res 2016;49.
11. Katz PO, Gerson LB, Vela MF. Guidelines for the diagnosis and management of gastroesophageal reflux disease. Am J Gastroenterol 2013;108:308–28 [quiz: 329].
12. Gyawali CP, Kahrilas PJ, Savarino E, et al. Modern diagnosis of GERD: the Lyon Consensus. Gut 2018;67:1351–62.
13. Hill LD, Kozarek RA. The gastroesophageal flap valve. J Clin Gastroenterol 1999; 28:194–7.
14. Cheng FK, Albert DM, Maydonovitch CL, et al. Categorization of patients with reflux symptoms referred for pH and impedance testing while off therapy. Clin Gastroenterol Hepatol 2015;13:867–73.
15. Park EY, Choi MG, Baeg M, et al. The value of early wireless esophageal pH monitoring in diagnosing functional heartburn in refractory gastroesophageal reflux disease. Dig Dis Sci 2013;58:2933–9.
16. Roman S, Gyawali CP, Savarino E, et al. Ambulatory reflux monitoring for diagnosis of gastro-esophageal reflux disease: Update of the Porto consensus and recommendations from an international consensus group. Neurogastroenterol Motil 2017;29:1–15.
17. Kessing BF, Bredenoord AJ, Smout AJ. Objective manometric criteria for the rumination syndrome. Am J Gastroenterol 2014;109:52–9.

18. Roman S, Holloway R, Keller J, et al. Validation of criteria for the definition of transient lower esophageal sphincter relaxations using high-resolution manometry. Neurogastroenterol Motil 2016;29(2).

19. Ren LH, Chen WX, Qian LJ, et al. Addition of prokinetics to PPI therapy in gastroesophageal reflux disease: a meta-analysis. World J Gastroenterol 2014;20: 2412–9.

20. Sifrim D, Castell D, Dent J, et al. Gastro-oesophageal reflux monitoring: review and consensus report on detection and definitions of acid, non-acid, and gas reflux. Gut 2004;53:1024–31.

21. Hillman L, Yadlapati R, Thuluvath AJ, et al. A review of medical therapy for proton pump inhibitor nonresponsive gastroesophageal reflux disease. Dis Esophagus 2017;30:1–15.

22. Yadlapati R, DeLay K. Proton pump inhibitor-refractory gastroesophageal reflux disease. Med Clin North Am 2019;103:15–27.

23. Bravi I, Woodland P, Gill RS, et al. Increased prandial air swallowing and postprandial gas-liquid reflux among patients refractory to proton pump inhibitor therapy. Clin Gastroenterol Hepatol 2013;11:784–9.

24. Herregods TV, Troelstra M, Weijenborg PW, et al. Patients with refractory reflux symptoms often do not have GERD. Neurogastroenterol Motil 2015;27:1267–73.

25. Rommel N, Tack J, Arts J, et al. Rumination or belching-regurgitation? Differential diagnosis using oesophageal impedance-manometry. Neurogastroenterol Motil 2010;22:e97–104.

26. Yadlapati R, Tye M, Roman S, et al. Postprandial high-resolution impedance manometry identifies mechanisms of nonresponse to proton pump inhibitors. Clin Gastroenterol Hepatol 2018;16:211–8.e1.

27. Kessing BF, Bredenoord AJ, Velosa M, et al. Supragastric belches are the main determinants of troublesome belching symptoms in patients with gastro-oesophageal reflux disease. Aliment Pharmacol Ther 2012;35:1073–9.

28. Kahrilas PJ, Bredenoord AJ, Fox M, et al. The Chicago classification of esophageal motility disorders, v3.0. Neurogastroenterol Motil 2015;27:160–74.

29. Fornari F, Bravi I, Penagini R, et al. Multiple rapid swallowing: a complementary test during standard oesophageal manometry. Neurogastroenterol Motil 2009; 21:718.

30. Pauwels A, Broers C, Van Houtte B, et al. A randomized double-blind, placebo-controlled, cross-over study using baclofen in the treatment of rumination syndrome. Am J Gastroenterol 2018;113:97–104.

Proton Pump Inhibitors
The Good, Bad, and Ugly

Felice Schnoll-Sussman, MD, Rachel Niec, MD, PhD,
Philip O. Katz, MD*

KEYWORDS

- PPIs • GERD • Acid control

KEY POINTS

- PPIs remain the medication of choice for GERD and multiple other clinical indications and are overwhelmingly safe drugs.
- PPIs are often used without clear indication, in excessive doses or duration.
- Multiple issues have been raised regarding potentially clinically important adverse events related to long-term use of PPIs.
- Balancing risk and benefits is paramount in managing patients who will clearly benefit from acid-suppressive therapy.

Some things change. Much remains the same. Proton pump inhibitors (PPIs) continue to be the mainstay of treatment of acid-related disease, especially gastroesophageal reflux disease (GERD). Without them many patients would experience a major decrement in their quality of life. PPIs are most frequently used for the acute and long-term management of GERD, being far superior to any other agent in this disease.[1] When needed, long-term therapy is effective in controlling symptoms, reducing recurrent erosive disease and peptic strictures, delaying progression of Barrett's esophagus to dysplasia, and maintaining complete remission of intestinal metaplasia (and dysplasia) after radiofrequency ablation for dysplasia in Barrett's esophagus. PPIs are effective, and often lifesaving, in prevention of gastrointestinal (GI) bleeding in patients on aspirin, dual antiplatelet therapy, nonsteroidal anti-inflammatory drugs, warfarin, and newer anticoagulants. Routine peptic ulcer disease is now rare and *Helicobacter pylori* substantially reduced in part because of the efficacy of this drug class. Furthermore, as a first-line mainstay of treatment of eosinophilic esophagitis, off label use of PPIs has been extremely valuable in management of this complex patient group.[2,3] (**Box 1**) When used according to clinical indication and in keeping with guidelines for use (using the lowest effective dose of PPIs needed to maintain symptom relief, treating only for indications and clinical situations in which they have shown clear

Division of Gastroenterology and Hepatology, Weill Cornell Medicine, 1315 York Avenue, New York City, NY 10021, USA
* Corresponding author.
E-mail address: Phk9009@med.cornell.edu

Gastrointest Endoscopy Clin N Am 30 (2020) 239–251
https://doi.org/10.1016/j.giec.2019.12.005
1052-5157/20/© 2019 Elsevier Inc. All rights reserved.

Box 1
Appropriate PPI indications: the good

PPI indications

Gastroesophageal reflux disease symptoms (trial of therapy)

Erosive esophagitis

Non-erosive reflux disease with abnormal ambulatory reflux monitoring

Barrett's esophagus

Peptic strictures

Eosinophilic esophagitis

Peptic ulcer disease

Helicobacter pylori eradication

Prevent GI bleeding in patients at risk on anticoagulants/antiplatelet therapy

Prevention of nonsteroidal anti-inflammatory drug complication

Hypersecretory states (Zollinger-Ellison syndrome)

Stress ulcer bleeding (short-term therapy)

---

benefit, and a clear recommendation to discontinue PPIs if they are not needed)[1] the safety profile of PPIs is excellent, with less than 1% to 2% of patients experiencing headache, nausea, abdominal pain, diarrhea, and requiring discontinuation of the medication.

However, there is little debate that the recommended prescribing guidelines are not always followed.[4] Therefore, PPIs are often overprescribed, sometimes in higher doses and for longer periods than indicated or required. This may be particularly true in patients treated empirically based on clinical presentation alone. Because this class of drugs was long believed to be essentially side effect free, there are many patients without clear initial or ongoing indication for use in whom attempts at dosage reduction or weaning have not been made. This has been highlighted by numerous reports of adverse events related to the use of PPIs, some of them potentially quite serious. **Table 1**. Those reports, principally case-control studies and meta-analyses, have been highly cited in the popular press and have raised questions about

Table 1
PPI adverse events: the bad and ugly

Older Risks of "Concern"	Other Potential PPI "Risks"	The Newest "Worries"
Fractures (FDA Class warning 2010, revised 2011)	Interstitial nephritis	Myocardial infarction
	Cardiac disease	Chronic kidney disease
Clopidogrel interaction (FDA warning 2009, different PPI labels)	Small intestinal bacterial overgrowth	Dementia
		Ischemic stroke
Clostridium difficile infection (FDA Class warning for enteric infections 2012)	Bacterial peritonitis	Asthma risk to child when used in first trimester
	Traveler's diarrhea	Early death
	Iron deficiency anemia	
Pneumonia	Rhabdomyolysis	
Magnesium deficiency (FDA Class warning 2011)		

the overuse and even appropriate use of PPIs. This has affected not only physicians' prescribing habits, but has also substantially increased patients' concerns about using these medications, particularly long-term.[5,6] Several Food and Drug Administration (FDA) warnings have resulted, including those related to long bone fractures, interaction with cladogram, enteric infections, and hypomagnesemia. More recently, concerns regarding PPIs and cardiovascular events have resurfaced, as have issues related to chronic kidney disease, dementia, cancer, and shortened lifespan. These studies report a statistical increase in adverse events associated with PPIs; however, they often lack sufficient statistical evidence to eliminate confounding variables and determine true causality. In many cases the adverse events are infrequent overall and do not fit with our clinical experience. Many articles suggest that the acid suppression associated with these drugs is responsible for multiple adverse events, whether related to absorption of electrolytes, vitamins and nutrients, changes in the gut microbiome or downstream effects on vascular integrity, or neurologic function. These concerns regarding acid suppression conflict with 2 clinical scenarios, pernicious anemia and vagotomy with antrectomy, in which documented achlorhydria occurs[7] and has not been conclusively associated with any of the reported adverse events with PPIs.

As with many reports relating to potential adverse effects of frequently prescribed medications, the reaction to the data has been widespread, particularly in the press, many times without careful consideration of the quality of the data, the methods of collection, and the magnitude of the effect of the adverse event. Clearly, it is paramount for optimal patient care for the physician and care provider to evaluate the available data with scrutiny and clinical perspective. The balance of this discussion will address the emerging literature of PPI adverse events and our recommendations for dealing with the conundrum of long-term management of acid-related disease. The major areas of concern will be highlighted and our considered recommendations for management presented.

MECHANISM OF ACTION AND ACID CONTROL

PPIs block the terminal step in acid production, blocking 70% to 80% of active potassium pumps on the apical membrane of gastric parietal cells and thus inhibiting hydrogen secretion into the gastric lumen; new pumps are constantly synthesized, a process that takes 36 to 96 hours. Although each of the available PPIs has subtly different binding capabilities, delayed-release PPIs in general provide maximal efficacy in control of intragastric pH when taken on an empty stomach 30 to 60 minutes before a meal as the drugs bind to actively secreting pumps. It is for this reason that these drugs are administered before the first meal of the day, or, when a second dose is needed, before the evening meal, rather than at bedtime. It is rare to see improved efficacy in acid control at higher doses than twice daily. PPI resistance is rarely if ever encountered, although substantial individual variability in acid control exists between patients, likely based on genetic polymorphism in the cytochrome p-450 system, which varies among ethnic groups. Although overall not a major clinical issue, this variability in acid control makes it difficult to determine a single optimal dosing regimen for all patients. As not all pumps are active at any given time, and thus a single dose of a PPI cannot inhibit all pumps and, therefore, will not "completely" inhibit all acid secretion. PPIs given once daily produce a wide range in the number of hours during which the intragastric pH is greater than 4, averaging about 12 hours, rarely going above 5 and much less reaching 7. Thus some hydrogen ion activity always remains. Intragastric pH rarely stays above 4 for more than 18 to 20 hours with any twice daily dosing regimen in H pylori-negative patients.[8,9] Achlorhydria is almost impossible to produce because of the constant pump turnover and continued synthesis of new pumps.[7] There is no substantive evidence that there are active proton pumps outside of the stomach.

CARDIOVASCULAR ISSUES

PPIs competitively inhibit activity of the CYP2C19 enzyme, the enzyme required for conversion of the prodrug, clopidogrel, to its active form. Thus, PPIs may reduce drug activation and potentially the desired antiplatelet effect. The clinical importance of this effect is unclear, but has resulted in the FDA warning physicians to be concerned about coprescribing PPIs in patients who take clopidogrel. Because of differences in CYP2C19 metabolism, omeprazole and esomeprazole seem to have the greatest effect, whereas lansoprazole, dexlansoprazole, pantoprazole, and, potentially, rabeprazole have less (if any) effect in vitro.[10–13]

A well-done meta-analysis reported significant increase in cardiovascular-related outcomes in patients who were on clopidogrel and also on PPIs.[14] In general the odds ratios (ORs) were low, less than 2, and as such subject to statistical error. Significant heterogeneity was observed between studies. When only randomized controlled trials were assessed, no statistically significant difference existed, suggesting that any potential interaction is not likely to be clinically significant.[14,15]

Attention has been paid to the alleged association between PPIs and an increased risk for myocardial infarction. One scientific basis for this concern comes from animal studies that show that PPIs increase asymmetric dimethyl arginine (ADMA) by binding to and inhibiting dimethylarginine dimethylaminohydrolase, which leads to decreased nitric oxide synthesis, which in turn is associated with increased vascular resistance and the promotion of inflammation and fibrosis.[16] Using a data-mining approach for pharmacovigilance of 2 large medical record databases there was a small but statistically significant increase with an OR of 1.16 (95% CI, 1.09, 1.24) for myocardial infarction (MI) in patients with GERD who were receiving PPIs.[17] However, comorbid diseases associated with cardiovascular disease, such as hypertension, obesity, and diabetes in patients with significant GERD were not reported. The same group of investigators conducted an open-label, crossover pilot study in humans—both healthy subjects and patients with coronary disease—to assess ADMA using a noninvasive device to measure endothelial function. They found that PPI use did not influence vascular endothelial function.[18]

Another retrospective study revealed an OR for MI of 1.13 (95% CI, 1.02, 1.26; $P = .02$) and a retrospective study assessing the role of PPI use before hospitalization for an infarction found an increased risk for MI in those exposed during the 7- and 14-day period preceding hospitalization.[19–21] The number needed to harm was approximately 4300. Overall the quality of these studies is difficult to assess and the ORs for harm extremely low.

Several more recent studies add to the difficulty in determining the potential for increase in cardiovascular disease associated with PPIs. A large study of greater than 6000 patients with diabetes who had a bare metal stent and received clopidogrel with or without PPIs for 90 days found no difference in acute coronary syndrome and readmission for revascularization (percutaneous coronary intervention or coronary artery bypass graft surgery) after 3, 6, and 12 months.[22] A systematic review of data from 16 studies, 8 of which were randomized controlled trials, found an increased risk of any adverse cardiovascular event with PPI in observational studies but not from randomized controlled trials (risk ratio = 0.89; 95% CI, 0.34–2.33; I2 0%, $P = .85$).[23] Furthermore, another meta-analysis of 4 randomized controlled trials and 8 controlled observational studies demonstrated statistical differences in major adverse cardio-vascular events in patients on PPIs; however, it conferred a reduction in risk of GI bleeding (OR = 0.58; 95% CI, 0.36–0.92; P = .022; I = 80.6%). There were no signif-icant differences in MI (OR = 1.03; 95% CI, 0.87–1.22; P = .742; I = 0%), cardiogenic death (OR = 1.09; 95% CI, 0.83–1.43; P = .526; I = 0%), or all-cause mortality (OR = 1.08; 95% CI, 0.93–1.25; P = .329; I = 0%).[24]

Overall, the balance of data from retrospective, large database studies favors an increased risk of potentially serious cardiac events; however, the ORs are low. When prospective randomized trials are considered these risks disappear. Two such studies are discussed below.

The Clopidogrel and the Optimization of Gastrointestinal Events Trial, was a high-quality randomized controlled trial. The effect of omeprazole 20 mg with or without clo-pidogrel 75 mg on a composite cardiovascular endpoint consisting of death from car-diovascular causes, nonfatal MI, revascularization, or ischemic stroke was measured. The event rate for the primary endpoint at 180 days was 4.9% in the omeprazole group and 5.7% in the placebo group (P = NS). The ORs for all cardiovascular events, MI, and revascularization were not significantly different between the 2 groups.[25]

A recent double-blind trial included 17,598 participants with stable cardiovascular and peripheral arterial disease randomly assigned patients to pantoprazole (40 mg daily, n = 8791) or placebo (n = 8807). Participants were also randomly assigned to rivaroxaban with aspirin, rivaroxaban, or aspirin alone. Data on development of pneu-monia, *Clostridium difficile* infection, other enteric infections, fractures, gastric atro-phy, chronic kidney disease, diabetes, chronic obstructive lung disease, dementia, cardiovascular disease, cancer, hospitalizations, and all-cause mortality were recorded every 6 months. Patients were followed up for a median of 3.01 years, a total of 53,152 patient-years of follow-up. There was no statistically significant difference between the pantoprazole and placebo groups in cardiovascular disease.[26] In fact there were no differences in any adverse events except for enteric infections (1.4% versus 1.0% in the placebo group; OR = 1.33; 95% CI, 1.01–1.75). There was a small increase in *C difficile* infection but only 13 events overall.[27]

Recommendation

Reconciling this large body of seemingly contradictory data into a clinical recommen-dation is difficult. What is clear is that the risk of major GI bleeding and its conse-quences outweigh what may be a potential risk of cardiovascular harm. A clear cause for cardiovascular harm does not as of this writing exist. Therefore, we do not restrict our use of PPIs in patients who need them, specifically those with risk for GI bleeding, a history of GI bleeding or with acid-related diseases who need PPIs for symptom relief. If there is concern either from the patient or care giver regarding potential interaction with clopidogrel then pantoprazole or dexlansoprazole can be considered. The data do not support any change in practice relative to concern for MI at this time.

DEMENTIA

One of the most recent of associations of PPIs with harm relate to 2 studies[26,28] revealing an association of PPI use with dementia. The basis for considering this relationship comes in part from the concern that PPIs may reduce absorption of vitamin B12, which may be associated with cognitive decline. The second is the finding in mice that PPIs can enhance beta-amyloid levels in the brains by affecting enzymes beta- and gamma-secretase. The first study was an analysis of data from a longitudinal prospective cohort of patients over the age of 75 years assessed with a series of neuropsychiatric interviews every 18 months in a primary care setting in Germany. The authors found a significant increase in hazard ratio (HR) (1.38) for incident dementia with PPI use. The second study from the same group used similar confounders to their previous study and found a similar HR (1.44) for incident dementia in patients using PPIs compared with those not. Occasional PPI use was associated with a modest increase in risk (HR = 1.16). Of note stroke, diabetes, age, and polypharmacy were associated with increased risk as were anticholinergic drugs. The PPI effect remained if these confounders were excluded.

A meta-analysis of 12 studies (8 cohort and 4 case-control) found that PPI use was not associated with dementia risk, with a pooled relative risk (RR) of 1.05 (95% CI, 0.96–1.15), P = .31. Subgroup analysis based on study design, sex (RR = 1.25; 95% CI, 0.97–1.60; P = .08), H2RA blockers (P = .93), and specifically for Alzheimer disease (RR = 1.00; 95% CI, 0.91–1.09; P = .93) also revealed no significant association between PPI use and dementia risk.[29]

A recent study using the prospectively collected nurse health study data showed no change in cognition after 9 years of PPI use.[30] Another recent study showed no increase in Alzheimer disease in patients exposed to PPIs[31]

Recommendation

Clearly this potential association raises considerable concerns so should not be dismissed. However, given the lack of a convincing potential cause of dementia and the balance of studies showing no increase in risk, we are not prepared to change practice patterns because of these data. Discussions with patients regarding adverse events, including the possibility of dementia, is a routine part of our practice.

RENAL DISEASE

There has long been an association of PPI use with acute interstitial nephritis, an infrequent but difficult to diagnose disease.[32–36] The disease is infrequent and the HR for the association with PPIs is also low (<2). Although accepted on the list of potential adverse events, the association of PPIs with chronic or end-stage renal disease has not been studied until recently. A series of investigations of large cohort databases found an increased HR for incident chronic kidney disease. Some association was found with length of use and dose (twice daily use produced HR higher than once daily). PPI use has been associated with a higher HR for chronic kidney disease than H2 receptor antagonists.[32] Another retrospective cohort study using a Veterans Affairs (VA) database found increased risk for increased serum creatinine, decreased glomerular filtration rate, and the development of end-stage renal disease in PPI users.[33] Increased risk was seen in those using PPIs for greater than 30 days but appeared to peak at 720 days. Multiple studies support an association between PPI use and patients with renal disease, all with similar odds or HRs and no plausible mechanism for the finding save for progression of interstitial nephritis.[34–36]

Recommendation: although the findings are of concern and definitely require further study, the associations are of insufficient strength to support regular monitoring on a large scale. It may, however, be prudent in patients at risk for chronic kidney disease to consider periodic monitoring of serum creatinine. In patients with known chronic kidney disease, PPIs should be prescribed with caution.

VITAMINS, MINERALS, AND FRACTURES

Concern has been raised that PPI therapy decreases the absorption of iron, calcium, and vitamin B12,[37–39] although clinical data are lacking. Hypomagnesemia has been reported, although the mechanism is not completely clear.[40,41] The best clinical evidence for lack of effect comes from the LOTUS and SOPRAN trials. Study patients were randomized to antireflux surgery or PPI therapy with esomeprazole 20 to 40 mg for ≥5 years (LOTUS) or omeprazole 20 to 40 mg for 10 to 12 years (SOPRAN). Levels of iron, calcium, and vitamin B12 remained constant in both the surgically and PPI-treated patients.[42]

Decrease in calcium absorption[43–45] and a subsequent decrease in bone mineral density (BMD) is the basis for believing that the association with fracture risk[46,47] is real. However, when carefully adjudicating case-control and cohort studies, the evidence for decreasing BMD is thin and fractures appear to be increased only in those with other risk factors (eg, smoking). A prospective analysis of the association between PPI use, BMD, and fracture risk in women reported no increase in the risk for hip fracture associated with current PPI use. There was, however, a slightly increased risk of spinal, forearm/wrist, and total fractures.[48] Meta-analyses of 10 observational studies reported a small risk for hip, vertebral, or wrist/forearm fractures, but again the ORs were less than ≤1.5.[49] Continuous PPI use over 5 years was not associated with accelerated BMD loss, osteoporosis of the hip or lumbar spine. No BMD loss was seen at any site during 5 and 10 years of follow-up.[50] A small but well-done study showed no evidence of loss of bone strength after 5 years continuous PPI use.[51] A very recent study showed no effect on measures of bone homeostasis in postmenopausal women.[52]

Recommendation

Given the data, we believe it is prudent to discuss the issues related to fractures with those patients at risk, particularly those who smoke. In patients with a history of fractures or known abnormalities in BMD consider referral to colleagues managing these issues. Restricting PPIs in patients for the sole purpose of avoiding fractures is not recommended. In patients requiring chronic high PPI doses we discuss alternatives: surgery or endoscopic antireflux therapy.

INFECTION

It is logical to think that PPIs could increase the risk of bacterial enteric infection by altering gut flora, many of which are responsive to pH. As with many plausible effects of gastric acid inhibition, this relationship has been difficult to substantiate. Associations with small intestinal bacterial overgrowth, traveler's diarrhea, and other enteric infections have been reported.[53–62] A more important relationship is that related to the potential risk of *C difficile* infection with PPI use.[62–67] The presumptive cause of this association is that PPIs decrease the gastric acid barrier or negatively affect the gut microbiome composition, preventing colonization resistance, and allowing for survival and/or passage of vegetative forms of the bacteria. PPIs may alter the composition and diversity of gut flora, favoring *C difficile* infection. In an FDA review, 23 of 28 observational studies showed a higher risk associated with PPI use. ORs varied between 1.4 and 2.8. A study showing a positive association between in-hospital PPI use and *C difficile* infection (OR = 1.96; 95% CI, 1.42, 2.72) also reported associations with antidepressants (OR = 2.99), anticonvulsants (OR = 2.02), antiplatelet agents (OR = 2.01), and osteoporosis medications (OR = 1.98). Most meta-analyses report ORs for the risk of infection less than 2, a level which is unlikely to represent causality.

Several studies report a risk of relapse with PPIs. Based on these data the FDA issued a class warning for the possibility of enteric infection and *C difficile* in patients on PPIs.

Recommendation

Continuing PPIs in instances where travel-related enteric infections are possible is a decision to be made between the patient and physician. No clear recommendation can be made save to be careful when prescribing PPIs to patients at risk for *C difficile*. Managing PPIs in patients at risk for or having *C difficile* infection must be individualized.

PERSPECTIVE

How are clinicians to modify their practice in light of the abundant yet conflicting data and the strong media push to reduce PPI usage. Crucial is the understanding that by all measures these associations, although statistically significant, are modest, and subject to statistical error. Although potentially serious, the events in question are unlikely to begin with PPI use and as such the absolute numbers needed to harm are extremely high. Although clearly smaller than the large database studies reporting associations with harm, prospective phase 3 trials, and several prospective cohort studies comparing PPI therapy to surgery have not reported concerns about renal or heart disease. One randomized VA study comparing medical to surgical therapy (no PPIs) reported an increase in cardiac-related death in the surgical arm (a finding dismissed as without basis). The most recent report, the randomized prospective trial mentioned above found no increase in adverse events (other than a small increase in enteric infections) with 3 years of continuous PPI use. Nevertheless, the body of evidence reporting the dangers of PPI use is large and continues to grow. Patients and physicians have discontinued medication with less than optimal information, sometimes with negative consequences. However, despite methodologic concerns and often small effect sizes, it is imprudent to ignore and dismiss these reported associations.

Therefore, we recommend the following: carefully assess the need for PPI therapy in patients with GERD. Consider objective evidence, such as early endoscopy and reflux testing, to firmly establish acid reflux as the culprit, especially in patients in whom the diagnosis is uncertain. Do not prescribe PPIs in hospitalized patients unless absolutely indicated (eg, GI bleeding and stress ulcer prophylaxis in high-risk patients) as they are often continued on discharge and seldom discontinued. Follow the guidelines! Prescribe empiric PPIs when the history dictates classic GERD symptoms. Have a low threshold for early work-up when dyspepsia is the primary symptoms and with any warning sign. In the absence of GERD complications, use the lowest effective dose or discontinue PPIs if possible. If PPIs are needed, discuss and consider alternatives, taking careful account of both success and adverse events (eg, surgery or endoscopic therapy for GERD), document your conversations (specifically those related to potential adverse effects) and involve patients in decision making. If PPIs are not indicated for symptom relief or prophylaxis, do not use them. If they are not working, look for alternative diagnoses and discontinue them. Limit increasing dosage in those without relief, and lastly consider switching PPIs once but no more than once.

Although practitioners may find it reassuring to see normal electrolytes, B12, urine analysis, creatinine, electrocardiograms, and BMD on routine regular monitoring, this may lead to false reassurance, is not cost effective, and further can come at a cost to the patient if abnormalities are incidentally discovered and not due to disease. Therefore, we do not recommend routine monitoring at this time. Perhaps most important, it is imperative to remind patients that medical management of GERD is not a substitute for a healthy lifestyle, including maintaining a normal body mass index, thoughtful attention to diet and exercise, moderation of alcohol intake, and avoidance of smoking.

Although the most recent 3-year prospective study is impressive for sure, we are unlikely to have prospective long-term data any time soon if at all. Therefore, well-designed studies that investigate intermediate markers of some of the disease endpoints (as has been done with dementia and bone disease) would be helpful. In particular, greater understanding of how PPIs affect the microbiome and whether changes in microbiota may influence some of the adverse events is paramount.

At this point, many questions exist regarding long-term use of PPIs. A drug class that has been a major boon to patients and physicians has come under fire, perhaps for several good reasons. Thus, it is crucial that we look carefully at the genesis of the data and at the magnitude of the risks that are being suggested and put them in context while we continue to conduct research and determine which, if any, of these adverse events are an actual concern.

DISCLOSURE

The authors have nothing to disclose.

REFERENCES

1. Katz PO, Gerson LB, Vela MF. Guidelines for the diagnosis and management of gastroesophageal reflux disease. Am J Gastroenterol 2013;108:308–28 [quiz: 329]. Detailed description of indications for diagnostic testing, description of esophageal physiologic tests, and use of diagnostic testing in making management recommendations.

2. Scarpignato C, Gatta L, Zullo A, et al. Effective and safe proton pump inhibitor therapy in acid-related diseases—a position paper addressing benefits and potential harms of acid suppression. BMC Med 2016;14:179. A valuable resource detailing state-of-the-art evidence for appropriate use of proton pump inhibitors.

3. Tan MC, El-Serag HB, Yu X, et al. Acid suppression medications reduce risk of oesophageal adenocarcinoma in Barrett's oesophagus: a nested case-control study in US male veterans. Aliment Pharmacol Ther 2018;48:469–77.

4. Vaezi MF, Yang YX, Howden CW. Complications of proton pump inhibitor therapy. Gastroenterology 2017;153(1):35–48. Detailed discussion of how to evaluate published literature addressing risks of long-term PPI therapy.

5. Kurlander JE, Kennedy JK, Rubenstein JH, et al. Patient's perceptions of proton pump inhibitor risks and attempts at discontinuation: a national survey. Am J Gastroenterol 2019;114:244–9.

6. Kurlander JE, Kolbe M, Rubenstein JH, et al. Internist's perceptions of proton pump inhibitor adverse effects and impact on prescribing practices: results of a nationwide survey. Gastroenterology Res 2018;11:11–7.

7. Wolfe MM, Sachs G. Acid suppression: optimizing therapy for gastroduodenal ulcer healing, gastroesophageal reflux disease, and stress-related erosive syndrome. Gastroenterology 2000;118(suppl):9–31.

8. Hatlebakk JG, Katz PO, Kuo B, et al. Nocturnal gastric acidity and acid breakthrough on different regimens of omeprazole 40 mg daily. Aliment Pharmacol Ther 1998;12:1235–40.

9. Katz P, Castell DO, Chen Y, et al. Esomeprazole 40 mg twice daily maintains intra-gastric pH > 4 more than 80% of a 24-hour time period. Am J Gastroenterol 2002; 97:520.

10. McGraw J, Waller D. Cytochrome P450 variations in different ethnic populations. Expert Opin Drug Metab Toxicol 2012;8(3):371–82.

11. Li XQ, Andersson TB, Ahlstrom M, et al. Comparison of inhibitory effects of the proton pump-inhbiting drugs omeprazole, esomeprazole, lansoprazole, panto-prazole, and rabeprazole on human cytochrome P450 activities. Drug Metab Dis-pos 2004;32(8):821–7.

12. Frelinger AL III, Lee RD, Mulford DJ, et al. A randomized, 2-period, crossover design study to assess the effects of dexlansoprazole, lansoprazole, esomepra-zole, and omeprazole on the steady-state pharmacokinetics and pharmacody-namics of clopidogrel in healthy volunteers. J Am Coll Cardiol 2012;59(14): 1304–11.

13. Hu W, Tong J, Kuang X, et al. Influence of proton pump inhibitors on clinical out-comes in coronary heart disease patients receiving aspirin and clopidogrel: a meta-analysis. Medicine (Baltimore) 2018;97(3):e9638.

14. Cardoso RN, Benjo AM, DiNicolantonio JJ, et al. Incidence of cardiovascular events and gastrointestinal bleeding in patients receiving clopidogrel with and without proton pump inhibitors: an updated meta-analysis. Open Heart 2015; 2(1):e000248.

15. Hsu PI, Lai KH, Liu CP. Esomeprazole with clopidogrel reduces peptic ulcer recurrence, compared with clopidogrel alone, in patients with atherosclerosis. Gastroenterology 2011;140(3):791–8.

16. Ghebremariam YT, LePendu P, Lee JC, et al. Unexpected effect of proton pump inhibitors: elevation of the cardiovascular risk factor asymmetric dimethylarginine. Circulation 2013;128(8):845–53.

17. Shah NH, LePendu P, Bauer-Mehren A, et al. Proton pump inhibitor usage and the risk of myocardial infarction in the general population. PLoS One 2015;10(6): e0124653.

18. Ghebremariam YT, Cooke JP, Khan F, et al. Proton pump inhibitors and vascular function: a prospective cross-over pilot study. Vasc Med 2015;20(4):309–16.

19. Charlot M, Ahlehoff O, Norgaard ML, et al. Proton-pump inhibitors are associated with increased cardiovascular risk independent of clopidogrel use: a nationwide cohort study. Ann Intern Med 2010;153(6):378–86.

20. Turkiewicz A, Vicente RP, Ohlsson H, et al. Revising the link between proton-pump inhibitors and risk of acute myocardial infarction - a case-crossover anal-ysis. Eur J Clin Pharmacol 2015;71(1):125–9.

21. Shih CJ, Chen YT, Ou SM, et al. Proton pump inhibitor use represents an indepen-dent risk factor for myocardial infarction. Int J Cardiol 2014;177(1):292–7.

22. Lee CW, Tsai FF, Su MI, et al. Effects of clopidogrel and proton pump inhibitors on cardiovascular events in patients with type 2 diabetes mellitus after bare metal stent implantation: a nationwide cohort study. Acta Cardiol Sin 2019;35(4): 402–11.

23. Batchelor R, Kumar R, Gilmartin-Thomas JFM, et al. Systematic review with meta-analysis: risk of adverse cardiovascular events with proton pump inhibitors inde-pendent of clopidogrel. Aliment Pharmacol Ther 2018;48(8):780–96.

24. Shiraev TP, Bullen A. Proton pump inhibitors and cardiovascular events: a sys-tematic review. Heart Lung Circ 2018;27(4):443–50.

25. Bhatt DL, Cryer BL, Contant CF, et al. Clopidogrel with or without omeprazole in coronary artery disease. N Engl J Med 2010;363(20):1909–17.

26. Haenisch B, von Holt K, WieseB, et al. Risk of dementia in elderly patients with the use of proton pump inhibitors. Eur Arch Psychiatry Clin Neurosci 2015;265(5): 419–28.

27. Moayyedi P, Eikelboom JW, Bosch J, et al. Safety of proton pump inhibitors based on a large, multi-year, randomized trial of patients receiving rivaroxaban or aspirin. Gastroenterology 2019;157(3):682–91.e2.

28. Gomm W, von Holt K, Thomé F, et al. Association of proton pump inhibitors with risk of dementia: a pharmacoepidemiological claims data analysis. JAMA Neurol 2016;73(4):410–4.

29. Wod M, Hallas J, Andersen K, et al. Lack of association between proton pump inhibitor use and cognitive decline. Clin Gastroenterol Hepatol 2018;16(5):681–9.

30. Lochhead P, Hagan K, Joshi AD, et al. Association between proton pump inhibitor use and cognitive function in women. Gastroenterology 2017;153(4):971–9.e4.

31. Taipale H, Tolppanen AM, Tiihonen M, et al. No association between proton pump inhibitor use and risk of Alzheimer's disease. Am J Gastroenterol 2017;112(12): 1802–8.

32. Larazus B, Chen Y, Wilson F, et al. Proton pump inhibitor use and the risk of chronic kidney disease. JAMA Intern Med 2016;176(2):238–46.

33. Xie Y, Bowe B, Li T, et al. Proton pump inhibitors and risk of incident CKD and progression to ESRD. J Am Soc Nephrol 2016;27:3153–63.

34. Yang Y, George KC, Shang WF, et al. Proton-pump inhibitors use, and risk of acute kidney injury: a meta-analysis of observational studies. Drug Des Devel Ther 2017;11:1291–9.

35. Klatte DCF, Gasparini A, Xu H, et al. Association between proton pump inhibitor use and risk of progression of chronic kidney disease. Gastroenterology 2017; 153(3):702–10.

36. Wijarnpreecha K, Thongprayoon C, Chesdachai S, et al. Associations of proton-pump inhibitors and H2 receptor antagonists with chronic kidney disease: a meta-analysis. Dig Dis Sci 2017;62(10):2821.

37. Termanini B, Gibril F, Sutliff VE, et al. Effect of long-term gastric acid suppressive therapy on serum vitamin B12 levels in patients with Zollinger-Ellison syndrome. Am J Med 1998;104(5):422–30.

38. den Elzen WP, Groeneveld Y, de RW, et al. Long-term use of proton pump inhibitors and vitamin B12 status in elderly individuals. Aliment Pharmacol Ther 2008; 27(6):491–7.

39. Qorraj-Bytyqi H, Hoxha R, Sadiku S, et al. Proton pump inhibitors intake and iron and vitamin B12 status: a prospective comparative study with a follow up of 12 months. Open Access Maced J Med Sci 2018;6(3):442–6.

40. Epstein M, McGrath S, Law F. Proton-pump inhibitors and hypomagnesemic hypoparathyroidism. N Engl J Med 2006;355(17):1834–6.

41. Koulouridis I, Alfayez M, Tighiouart H, et al. Out-of-hospital use of proton pump inhibitors and hypomagnesemia at hospital admission: a nested case-control study. Am J Kidney Dis 2013;62(4):730–7.

42. Attwood SE, Ell C, Galmiche JP, et al. Long-term safety of proton pump inhibitor therapy assessed under controlled, randomised clinical trial conditions: data from the SOPRAN and LOTUS studies. Aliment Pharmacol Ther 2015;41(11): 1162–74.

43. O'Connell MB, Madden DM, Murray AM, et al. Effects of proton pump inhibitors on calcium carbonate absorption in women: a randomized crossover trial. Am J Med 2005;118(7):778–81.

44. Kopic S, Geibel JP. Gastric acid, calcium absorption, and their impact on bone health. Physiol Rev 2013;93(1):189–268.

45. Wright MJ, Sullivan RR, Gaffney-Stomberg E, et al. Inhibiting gastric acid production does not affect intestinal calcium absorption in young, healthy individuals: a randomized, crossover, controlled clinical trial. J Bone Miner Res 2010;25(10):2205–11.

46. Yang YX, Lewis JD, Epstein S, et al. Long-term proton pump inhibitor therapy and risk of hip fracture. JAMA 2006;296(24):2947–53.

47. Corley DA, Kubo A, Zhao W, et al. Proton pump inhibitors and histamine-2 receptor antagonists are associated with hip fractures among at-risk patients. Gastroenterology 2010;139(1):93–101.

48. Gray SL, LaCroix AZ, Larson J, et al. Proton pump inhibitor use, hip fracture, and change in bone mineral density in postmenopausal women: results from the Women's Health Initiative. Arch Intern Med 2010;170(9):765–71.

49. Ngamruengphong S, Leontiadis GI, Radhi S, et al. Proton pump inhibitors and risk of fracture: a systematic review and meta-analysis of observational studies. Am J Gastroenterol 2011;106(7):1209–18 [quiz: 1219].

50. Targownik LE, Lix LM, Leung S, et al. Proton-pump inhibitor use is not associated with osteoporosis or accelerated bone mineral density loss. Gastroenterology 2010;138(3):896–904.

51. Targownik LE, Goertzen AL, Luo Y, et al. Long-term proton pump inhibitor use is not associated with changes in bone strength and structure. Am J Gastroenterol 2017;112(1):95–101.

52. Hansen KE, Nieves JW, Nudurupati S, et al. Dexlansoprazole and esomeprazole do not affect bone homeostasis in healthy postmenopausal women. Gastroenterology 2019;156:926–34.

53. Leonard J, Marshall JK, Moayyedi P. Systematic review of the risk of enteric infection in patients taking acid suppression. Am J Gastroenterol 2007;102(9):2047–56.

54. Doorduyn Y, Van Den Brandhof WE, Van Duynhoven YT, et al. Risk factors for *Salmonella enteritidis* and *Typhimurium* (DT104 and non-DT104) infections in the Netherlands: predominant roles for raw eggs in *enteritidis* and sandboxes in *Typhimurium* infections. Epidemiol Infect 2006;134(3):617–26.

55. Freeman R, Dabrera G, Lane C, et al. Association between use of proton pump inhibitors and non-typhoidal salmonellosis identified following investigation into an outbreak of *Salmonella* Mikawasima in the UK, 2013. Epidemiol Infect 2015;144(5):968–75.

56. Doorduyn Y, Van Den Brandhof WE, Van Duynhoven YT, et al. Risk factors for indigenous *Campylobacter jejuni* and *Campylobacter coli* infections in the Netherlands: a case-control study. Epidemiol Infect 2010;138(10):1391–404.

57. DuPont HL, Formal SB, Hornick RB, et al. Pathogenesis of *Escherichia coli* diarrhea. N Engl J Med 1971;285(1):1–9.

58. Bavishi C, DuPont HL. Systematic review: the use of proton pump inhibitors and increased susceptibility to enteric infection. Aliment Pharmacol Ther 2011;34(11–12):1269–81.

59. Diemert DJ. Prevention and self-treatment of traveler's diarrhea. Clin Microbiol Rev 2006;19(3):583–94.

60. Juckett G. Prevention and treatment of traveler's diarrhea. Am Fam Physician 1999;60(1):119–24.

61. Schwille-Kiuntke J, Mazurak N, Enck P. Systematic review with meta-analysis: post-infectious irritable bowel syndrome after travellers' diarrhoea. Aliment Pharmacol Ther 2015;41(11):1029–37.

62. Dalton BR, Lye-Maccannell T, Henderson EA, et al. Proton pump inhibitors increase significantly the risk of *Clostridium difficile* infection in a low-endemicity, non-outbreak hospital setting. Aliment Pharmacol Ther 2009;29(6):626–34.

63. Janarthanan S, Ditah I, Adler DG, et al. *Clostridium difficile*-associated diarrhea and proton pump inhibitor therapy: a meta-analysis. Am J Gastroenterol 2012; 107(7):1001–10.

64. Zacharioudakis IM, Zervou FN, Pliakos EE, et al. Colonization with toxinogenic *C. difficile* upon hospital admission, and risk of infection: a systematic review and meta-analysis. Am J Gastroenterol 2015;110(3):381–90.

65. Seto CT, Jeraldo P, Orenstein R, et al. Prolonged use of a proton pump inhibitor reduces microbial diversity: implications for *Clostridium difficile* susceptibility. Microbiome 2014;2:42.

66. Jump RL, Pultz MJ, Donskey CJ. Vegetative *Clostridium difficile* survives in room air on moist surfaces and in gastric contents with reduced acidity: a potential mechanism to explain the association between proton pump inhibitors and *C. difficile*-associated diarrhea? Antimicrob Agents Chemother 2007;51(8): 2883–7.

67. Tariq R, Singh S, Gupta A, et al. Association of gastric acid suppression with recurrent clostridium difficile infection: a systematic review and meta-analysis. JAMA Intern Med 2017;177(6):784–91.

Nonablative Radiofrequency Treatment for Gastroesophageal Reflux Disease (STRETTA)

Piotr Sowa, MD, Jason B. Samarasena, MD*

KEYWORDS

- Stretta • Radiofrequency energy • Gastroesophageal reflux disease
- GERD in altered anatomy

KEY POINTS

- Stretta is indicated for patients with GERD who have a contraindication to medical therapy, or have concerns regarding the long-term side effects of the PPI class of medications, and either do not qualify or refuse surgical options for the treatment of GERD.
- Stretta has an excellent safety profile.
- The underlying mechanism of action of Stretta is unclear and controversial but likely does not involved tissue fibrosis.
- Optimal candidates for Stretta seem to be patients with hiatal hernia or diaphragmatic hiatus less than 2 cm, patients with typical GERD symptoms who are partially responsive to PPI therapy, and who are predominantly upright refluxers.

INTRODUCTION

Gastroesophageal reflux disease (GERD) is one of the most common digestive tract ailments and is the most frequent outpatient diagnosis in the United States.[1] Patients suffer from an impairment in quality of life, presenting with such symptoms as heartburn, regurgitation, or dysphagia. Proton pump inhibitors (PPIs) have made great improvements in symptoms of GERD but can provide incomplete relief of symptoms in a large proportion of patients. This partial response may be because PPIs do not address an incompetent sphincter valve or prevent reflux itself. In addition, some patients are reluctant to commit to lifelong therapy on PPIs in light of potential concerns of the complications of long-term PPI use, such as bone fracture, pneumonia, and enteric infections.[2–4] As a consequence, patients have started to seek alternative means of treating their GERD if their quality of life is compromised.[5] Refractory GERD, which is defined by less than 50% improvement of reflux symptoms including heartburn despite at least 12 weeks of double-dose PPI therapy,[6] entails that there is

University of California – Irvine, Orange, CA, USA
* Corresponding author. 300 City Boulevard West, Orange, CA 92868.
E-mail address: jsamaras@uci.edu

Gastrointest Endoscopy Clin N Am 30 (2020) 253–265
https://doi.org/10.1016/j.giec.2019.12.006
1052-5157/20/© 2019 Elsevier Inc. All rights reserved.

clinically significant impairment in the quality of life because of episodes of reflux despite PPI therapy. It is notable that such refractory GERD symptoms may not always reflect the acidity of the refluxate but rather the increased refluxate volume, esophageal compliance, and individual sensitivity to acid.[7,8] Sustained GERD also predisposes many patients to more serious adverse events, such as erosive esophagitis, Barrett's esophagus, and esophageal adenocarcinoma[9]

Laparoscopic fundoplication is currently considered to be the most robust operation for the treatment of reflux disease, but this operation does carry some significant side effects. Among the most common include dysphagia, gas and bloating, and an inability to belch. Other disadvantages include the invasive nature of laparoscopic fundoplication, the risk of a surgical procedure, and the permanent anatomic alteration of the gastroesophageal junction (GEJ). These factors may account for the decreasing number of surgical fundoplications performed in recent years.[10]

For the patient with refractory GERD, with surgical fundoplication, there is a steep rise in the invasiveness of therapy after PPI failure. As a result this has created a "therapeutic gap" between medical and surgical therapy. This has resulted in significant research for developing endoscopic procedures to alleviate symptoms of refractory GERD. A large number of procedures and techniques have failed in this arena for several reasons including a poor understanding of GERD physiology, lack of high-quality evidence, severe adverse events, and unsuccessful business planning. One of the endoscopic procedures for the management of GERD in the United States is the Stretta (Restech, Houston, TX) system. This procedure uses radiofrequency (RF) energy, which is applied to the muscles of the lower esophageal sphincter (LES) and the gastric cardia resulting in an improvement of reflux symptoms. This review evaluates the most recent data on the efficacy, mechanisms of action, and safety of this procedure.

PROCEDURAL TECHNIQUE

The Stretta system (Restech, Houston, TX) is comprised of a four-channel RF generator (**Fig. 1**) and single-use RF energy catheters (**Fig. 2**). At the start of the procedure, the patient is positioned in a left lateral decubitus position. The return electrode pad is positioned on the patient's right midscapular region, off the midline.

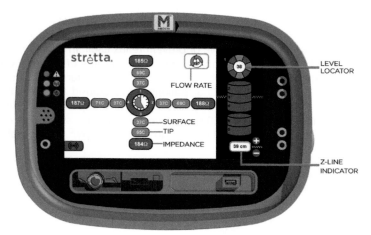

Fig. 1. RF generator for Stretta procedure. (© 2020 Restech | Mederi-RF.)

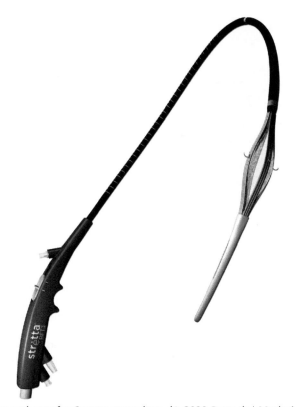

Fig. 2. Single-use catheter for Stretta procedure. (© 2020 Restech | Mederi-RF.)

A standard esophagogastroduodenoscopy (EGD) procedure is first performed, with careful inspection, measurement, and guidewire placement to confirm the location and depth of the patient's squamocolumnar junction (SCJ). The Stretta procedure catheter is introduced over the guidewire into the esophagus, advanced to 1 cm proximal to the SCJ. The generator is then switched from standby to ready mode. Suction is attached to the catheter. The balloon basket assembly is then inflated via the syringe and pressure release valve (to prevent overinflation) and four nitinol needle electrodes (22 gauge, 5.5 mm) are extended fully into the muscular layer of the esophageal wall (**Fig. 3**). Pressing on the foot pedal then engages the RF generator to deliver pure sine-wave energy (465 kHz, 2–5 W per channel, 80 V maximum at 100–800 Ω) into the LES muscle for 60 seconds, resulting in a thermal reaction (**Fig. 4**). Following this treatment cycle, the needles are retracted and the balloon is deflated. Pulling the catheter back to 25 cm, the catheter is then rotated 45° to the right and then readvanced back into position 1 cm from the SCJ. The balloon is reinflated, and the needles are extended as before. RF energy is delivered to four additional points (**Fig. 5**).

This entire process is repeated at three additional levels: at 0.5 cm above the SCJ, at the SCJ, and 0.5 cm below the SCJ up the esophagus. After this part of the procedure, it is our practice to remove the catheter and inspect the area thus far treated with the endoscope. We look for evidence of cautery marks at the expected levels.

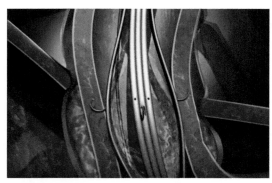

Fig. 3. Four nitinol needle electrodes engaged in the muscular layer of the esophageal wall. (© 2020 Restech | Mederi-RF.)

The guidewire is then reintroduced and the catheter is advanced into the stomach. The guidewire is then removed and the balloon is inflated to 25 mL, and withdrawn until it is snug to the hiatus. The needles are extended, and a 60-second treatment cycle is completed. The needles then get retracted, and the catheter is advanced into the stomach and rotated 30° to the right. Pulling back against the hiatus again, another treatment cycle is completed. Finally, a third treatment cycle is performed at 30° to the left of the original treatment cycle.

For the last treatment level, the catheter is again advanced into the stomach, and the balloon is inflated to 22 mL. The catheter is then withdrawn until the balloon is again snug at the hiatus. A similar pattern of three treatment cycles is again performed at this level (**Fig. 6**).

Throughout the procedure, there is constant chilled irrigation of water (not saline) applied to the esophageal and cardiac mucosa to prevent undesirable complications of mucosal injury, such as ulcerations or strictures.

Following completion of the procedure, the balloon is deflated and the catheter is removed. We recommend a post-procedure EGD to carefully inspect the treatment sites and to confirm no immediate complications related to the procedure. We are also specifically looking for evidence of cautery marks within the cardia and a swelling of the valve on a retroflexed view.

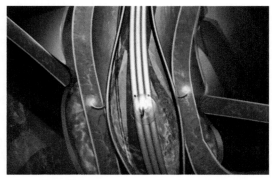

Fig. 4. Thermal reaction of the first treatment cycle of Stretta procedure. (© 2020 Restech | Mederi-RF.)

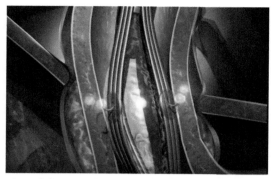

Fig. 5. Thermal reaction of the second treatment cycle, offset by 45° from first cycle. (© 2020 Restech | Mederi-RF.)

STRETTA EFFICACY

The Stretta procedure has been shown to be effective in numerous studies. Liu and colleagues[11] conducted a 12-month follow-up of 90 patients undergoing the Stretta procedure and found that at 2 months of follow-up, the onset of GERD symptom relief was 70% to 16.7% at 2 to 6 months, respectively. The mean GERD health-related quality-of-life questionnaire (HRQL) score was 25.6 at baseline, which dropped to 7.3 at 6 months ($P<.01$), reaching 8.1 at 12 months ($P<.01$). The authors report that the mean heartburn score was 3.3 at baseline, dropping to 1.2 at 12 months ($P<.05$). They add that the percentage of patients with satisfactory GERD control improved from 31.1% at baseline to 86.7% after the Stretta procedure, with patient satisfaction improving from 1.4 at baseline to 4.0 at 12 months ($P<.01$). Medication use also decreased significantly from 100% of patients using PPIs to 76.7% of patients eliminating use of medications or only as needed at 12 months. The authors have also demonstrated that after 6 months post-Stretta, improvement of endoscopic grade of esophagitis in 33 of the 41 patients occurred. All patients either had no erosions or only mild erosive disease (grade A).

A nonrandomized, prospective, multicenter study including 118 patients with chronic heartburn and/or regurgitation requiring daily antisecretory medication and exhibiting pathologic esophageal acid exposure, a sliding hiatal hernia less than or equal to 2 cm, and esophagitis less than or equal to grade 2 was performed.[12] At

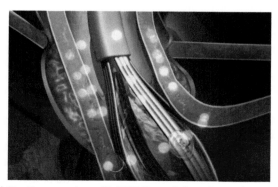

Fig. 6. Completed Stretta procedure. (© 2020 Restech | Mederi-RF.)

12 months, there were improvements in the median heartburn score from 4 to 1 (P = .0001), GERD score from 27 to 9 (P = .0001), satisfaction from 1 to 4 (P = .0001), mental Short Form (SF)-36 from 46.3 to 55.4 (P<.0001), and physical Short Form-36 from 40.9 to 53.1 (P = .0001). PPI requirement dropped from 88.1% to 30% of patients. Furthermore, esophageal acid exposure improved significantly from 10.2% to 6.4% (P = .0001). Eighteen of the patients agreed to undergo esophageal manometry: there was no significant change in any esophageal motility parameter, although there seemed to be a reduction in the number of transient LES relaxations (tLESRs).

Corley and colleagues[13] conducted a randomized, sham-controlled study using Stretta. In this study, 64 GERD patients were randomized to either having Stretta (n = 35) or a sham procedure (n = 29) done. Primary outcomes were reflux symptoms and quality of life. At the 6-month follow-up, Stretta significantly and substantially improved patients' heartburn symptoms (mean decrease, -1.6 [95% confidence interval (CI), -1.1 to -2.2] vs -0.6 [95% CI, 0.1 to -1.2]; P = .01) and quality of life (GERD-HRQL scores mean decrease, -13 points [95% CI, -9 to -17] vs -3 points [95% CI, -8 to 2]; P = .003). More Stretta versus sham patients were considered treatment responders with greater than 50% improvement in the GERD-HRQL score (61% vs 30%; P = .03) and without daily heartburn symptoms (61% vs 33%; P = .05). The active treatment group's improvements in symptoms and GERD-HRQL were sustained at the 12-month follow-up.

Coron and colleagues[14] conducted a prospective, randomized trial comparing the Stretta procedure with PPI therapy in patients who are PPI-dependent. In the Stretta group, 18/20 patients stopped (n = 3) or decreased (n = 15) PPI use compared with 8/16 in the PPI group (P = .01). None of the control patients could stop PPI usage. HRQL scores between the two groups were not different. There was no significant change noted in the esophageal acid exposure between baseline and 6 months following Stretta.

Some of the longer follow-up studies published have been to 48-month of follow-up after the Stretta procedure.[15–17] Noar and Lofti-Emran report that out of the 109 patients they treated with the Stretta procedure, heartburn scores decreased from a mean of 3.67 to 1.18 (standard deviation [SD], 1.28; P<.001), total heartburn score based on the GERD-HRQL decreased from a mean of 27.8 to 7.1 (SD, 8.42; P<.001), and patient satisfaction also improved from a mean of 1.4 to 3.8 (SD, 1.09; P<.001).[16] In the same population, medication usage decreased significantly from baseline, because 100% of patients were on a daily PPI to 75% of patients demonstrating elimination of medications or only as need use at 48 months. Reymunde and Santiago report similar results with GERD symptom scores improved from a mean of 2.7 at baseline to 0.3 at 36 months, then 0.6 at 48 months.[17] The mean quality of life scores improved from 2.4 at baseline, to 4.6 at 36 months, then 4.3 at 48 months (P<.001). A total of 90.2% of the patients on PPI or H_2 receptor antagonists before the Stretta procedure reduced their medication to none at all; 88.75% had complete elimination or reduction in their use of PPIs. Dughera and colleagues[15] contend that mean heartburn and GERD-HRQL scores decreased significantly at 48 months (P = .001 and P = .003, respectively). In addition, 72.3% of patients were completely off PPIs, although 14% of patients were still using occasional antacids, but none of them of a weekly basis.

Several studies have shown durability of the Stretta procedure with follow-up over an 8-and 10-year period. In the study with an 8-year follow-up,[18] 26 patients who underwent the Stretta procedure underwent clinical evaluation by upper endoscopy, esophageal pressure, and pH studies. The authors found a significant decrease in heartburn and GERD HRQL scores at 4 years ($P = .001$) and at 8 years ($P = .003$), and increase of quality of life scores at each control time (mental SF-36 and physical SF-36, $P = .001$). After 4 years, 80.7% of patients were completely off PPIs ($P = .0001$). After 8 years, 76.9% of patients were completely off PPIs ($P = .0001$). Median LES pressure did not improve at 4 and 8 years. Mean esophageal acid exposure significantly improved at 4 years ($P = .001$) but returned to baseline at 8 years. The authors conclude that Stretta is a durable procedure that allows patients to decrease intake of PPIs.

Noar and colleagues[19] published their results on Stretta after a 10-year follow-up. Using an intent-to-treat analysis, the authors prospectively assessed 217 patients with medically refractory GERD before and after Stretta. The primary outcome measure was the normalization of the GERD HRQL score in 70% or greater of patients at the end of the 10 years. Secondary outcomes were 50% reduction or elimination of PPIs and 60% or greater improvement in satisfaction at 10 years. At 10 years, the primary outcome was achieved in 72% of patients (95% CI, 65–79). For secondary outcomes, a 50% or greater in reduction of PPI usage occurred in 64% of patients, with 41% of patients eliminating PPI usage entirely. A 60% or greater increase in satisfaction occurred in 54% of patients. The authors conclude that after a 10-year follow-up, Stretta persists to be a durable procedure.

A meta-analysis published in 2012 by Perry and colleagues[20] of 18 studies and 1441 patients concluded the following: Stretta (1) is effective in symptom relief of GERD, (2) is safe and well-tolerated, and (3) significantly reduces acid exposure to the esophagus but does not consistently normalize pH. This last point is of note in that in up to 50% of GERD patients symptomatically controlled with PPIs, PPIs did not normalize pH.[21] Thus, pH normalization may not necessarily be an important clinical end point that needs to be applied to the Stretta procedure or other antireflux procedures/interventions.

In cases where a single Stretta procedure does not produce long-lasting effects, the procedure may be repeated. Aziz and colleagues[22] report a prospective randomized trial of sham, single-dose Stretta, and double-dose Stretta. Thirty-six patients were followed: in group A, 12 patients underwent a single Stretta procedure; in group B, 12 patients underwent a sham Stretta procedure; and in group C, 12 patients underwent a single Stretta procedure followed by a repeat Stretta if GERD-HRQL was not 75% improved after 4 months. Results showed a significant improvement in heartburn and regurgitation symptoms at 12 months in all groups, with improvement from baseline numerically but not statistically superior for group C compared with group A. That being said, no patients in group B normalized their HRQL scores, whereas two patients in group A normalized their HRQL scores and seven in group C (double Stretta vs single Stretta, $P<.05$; double Stretta vs sham, $P<.05$). As with the previous studies noted, at 12 months 50% of the patients were off all GERD-related medications, the remaining having a drop in their PPI doses ($P<.01$). A total of 16.6% of patients completely went off all GERD-related medications by 12 months in the single Stretta group.

Despite the positive results of the studies cited previously, there has still been controversy on the durability of the Stretta procedure. Dundon and colleagues[23] report that the Stretta procedure does not provide long-term symptom relief. In their study, of the 32 patients who completed the 6-month follow-up survey, 19 patients were considered to be treatment failures, 12 of them undergoing Nissen fundoplication and 7 undergoing Roux-en-Y gastric bypass surgery. Mean follow-up time was 53 months, ranging from 36 to 68 months. In this study, 59% of the patients eventually proceeded to antireflux surgery, with only 6% achieving durable symptomatic control without PPIs beyond

3 years. The authors also noted that those individuals who eventually proceeded to anti-reflux surgery showed significantly higher pre-Stretta heartburn severity than those who were responsive to the Stretta procedure. The discrepancy in these authors' findings may be attributable to the fact that all of the patients had already been referred to surgery and were therefore likely to be more severe cases.

A recent systematic review and meta-analysis conducted by Lipka and colleagues[24] also contended that there is no evidence for the efficacy of Stretta. This paper came out as a response to the strong recommendation for Stretta for the treatment of GERD in carefully selected patients put forth by the Society of American Gastrointestinal and Endoscopic Surgeons, which was in part based on the findings in the meta-analysis published by Perry and colleagues.[20] In this review and meta-analysis, the authors collected data from four trials, three trials comparing Stretta with sham and one comparing Stretta with PPI therapy, studying 153 patients. Lipka and colleagues[24] indicate that the quality of evidence was very low and that the pooled results show no difference between Stretta and sham or Stretta and management with PPI in patients with GERD. The authors conclude that Stretta does not produce significant changes compared with sham therapy with regard to time spent at a pH less than 4, LES pressure, ability to stop PPIs, or HRQL. Society of American Gastrointestinal and Endoscopic Surgeons responded to Lipka and colleagues[24] stating that on careful review of their data there were in fact improvements regarding quality of life, percent off PPI, and LES pressure but because only a small number of Stretta trials were included the results were not statistically significant.

A systematic review and meta-analysis published by Fass and colleagues[25] published in 2017 confirmed that the Stretta procedure significantly improves subjective and objective clinical end points and should be considered as a viable option in the management of GERD. Twenty-eight studies representing 2468 unique Stretta patients were included in the meta-analysis. The data showed that the Stretta procedure improved HRQL score by -14.6 (-16.48 to -12.73; $P<.001$) and pooled heartburn standardized score by -1.53 (-1.97 to -1.09; $P<.001$). PPI use was stopped in 51% of Stretta patients at follow-up, erosive esophagitis incidence was reduced by 24%, and esophageal acid exposure was reduced by a mean of -3.01 (-3.72 to -2.30; $P<.001$). Despite reduction in acid reflux, the procedure had no effect on LES basal pressure measurements post-Stretta by a mean of 1.73 (-0.29 to -3.74) mm Hg. This study included a large number of studies with a wide range of patient populations, health care systems, investigators, and a high number of research subjects and the authors argue that it represents real-world effectiveness of the Stretta procedure.

Overall, the Stretta procedure has been shown to be effective in multiple separate clinical studies and a large meta-analysis. Stretta has been shown to achieve a high rate of GERD symptom control over and above PPI therapy, and a decrease or altogether elimination of GERD medication has been demonstrated.

INDICATIONS AND PATIENT SELECTION FOR STRETTA

Stretta is indicated for patients with GERD who have a contraindication to medical therapy, or have concerns regarding the long-term side effects of the PPI class of medications, and either do not qualify or refuse surgical options for the treatment of GERD. Preoperative preparation includes a diagnostic EGD to evaluate for structural abnormalities, such as hiatal hernia; the presence of GEJ weakness (Hill grading system); and to characterize the presence of sequelae of GERD, such as esophagitis, Barrett's esophagus, or strictures/rings. For nonerosive reflux disease, further testing with 48-hour wireless pH monitoring is recommended to confirm the presence of pathologic reflux. High-resolution esophageal manometry testing should be performed to rule out the presence of achalasia or other esophageal motility disorders.

The presence of a hiatal hernia greater than 2 cm or a diaphragmatic hiatus greater than 2 cm makes for a poor candidate for the Stretta procedure. Patients with Hill grade 3 or 4 are also not appropriate for Stretta. In fact, in our experience the best candidates for Stretta are those with little to no anatomic abnormality of the GEJ as seen on EGD. The mechanism of action for reflux in these patients is likely driven by a functional issue of the valve including increased frequency of tLESRs. Typically, these patients are upright daytime refluxers as evidenced on an ambulatory pH monitoring study.

Failure to respond to medical therapy portends poorer responses to antireflux procedures. First evaluate for alternative causes of their symptoms, including hypersensitive esophagus and functional heartburn. Achalasia or incomplete LES relaxation in response to swallow must be evaluated for before therapy considerations, because of the risk of worsening these conditions following therapy.

STRETTA IN ALTERED ANATOMY

There are limited treatment options for GERD in patients with altered anatomy. GERD occurs de novo or intensifies after laparoscopic sleeve gastrectomy resulting in reflux symptoms. A retrospective study published by Khidir and colleagues[26] showed that post laparoscopic sleeve gastrectomy patients with pathologic GERD did not have significant improvement in GERD symptoms following Stretta procedure. In this study GERD was confirmed by 24-hour pH monitoring, presence of esophagitis on endoscopy, or presence of reflux on barium imaging. PPI dosage and GERD-HRQL questionnaire were reviewed at 0, 3, and 6 months. Mean HRQL scores were 42.7 ± 8.9 pre-Stretta and 41.8 ± 11 at 6 months ($P = .8$). At 6 months 66.7% of patients were not satisfied with the procedure; however, 20% of patients were able to stop PPI use.

Stretta has been shown to reduce gastroesophageal reflux patient-reported outcomes in a failed laparoscopic Nissen fundoplication (LNF) cohort. Noar and colleagues[27] compared long-term patient-reported outcomes of Stretta in refractory patients with and without previous LNH. In this prospective study, 18 GERD-refractory LNF patients and 81 standard anatomy patients were followed 10 years following Stretta procedure; GERD-HRQL, patient satisfaction scores, and daily medication requirements were assessed. The refractory LNH subset demonstrated median improvement in GERD-HRQL, satisfaction, and medication use at all follow-up time points greater than 6 months to 10 years. At 10 years, median GERD-HRQL decreased from 36 to 7 ($P<.001$), satisfaction increased from 1 to 4 ($P<.001$), and medication score decreased from 7 to 6 ($P = .040$). No significant difference was observed between refractory LNF and standard refractory GERD subsets at any follow-up time points greater than 6 months to 10 years ($P>.05$) following Stretta. In this refractory LNF cohort, the Stretta procedure resulted in sustained improvement in GERD symptoms with equivalent outcomes to non-LNF patients. Stretta seems to be a viable option in post-LNF patients who continue to have refractory GERD symptoms and who do not wish or do not qualify for repeat invasive surgery.

STRETTA MECHANISMS OF ACTION

There has been some debate as to how the Stretta procedure produces its effects. Some have posed that RF energy causes a limited coagulative necrosis of the tissue, which is healed by fibrosis.[28,29] However, because the mucosal temperature is kept well under the accepted level of tissue ablation (100°C), it is unlikely that tissue destruction followed by fibrosis occurs.[30] One animal study examined the effect of the Stretta procedure to the porcine GEJ and its effect on LES pressure and gastric yield pressure.[31] In this study, 20 pigs underwent esophageal manometry and endoscopic injection of 100 units of botulinum toxin into the LES. The animals were then randomized to either receive Stretta (n = 13) or no further intervention (control animals, n = 7) after 1 week. At Week 9, the animals underwent endoscopy, manometry, and gastric yield pressure determination. The control animals experienced a mean LES pressure decline by 3.7 ± 2.6 mm Hg (P = .03), whereas the animals receiving Stretta declined by 0.97 ± 5.8 mm Hg (P = .29). Additionally, the mean gastric yield pressure was 24.9 ± 8.2 mm Hg (control animals), versus 43.4 ± 10.7 mm Hg in the Stretta group (P = .0007). The authors concluded that Stretta reversed most of the LES pressure reduction accomplished with botulinum toxin injection and increased gastric yield pressure by 75% when compared with the control subjects.

Another animal study explored the effect of Stretta to the gastric cardia on the triggering of tLESRs and GERD.[32] This study was done on 13 dogs, 11 receiving Stretta and 2 control animals. Esophageal motility and pH were measured for 1 hour after a standard liquid meal and air infusion; this was repeated before and 3 months after the Stretta procedure. At the seventh month, histologic evaluation of the GEJ was performed. Stretta was found to significantly reduce the frequency of tLESRs from median of 4.0 (interquartile range, 3.0–6.75) per hour to median of 3.0 (interquartile range, 2.0–3.0) per hour (P<.05). Also, there was a significant reduction in acid reflux episodes and esophageal acid exposure. Additionally, there was a 63% increase in the wall thickness of the gastric cardia when compared with that in the two control dogs, but no histopathologic abnormalities in the esophageal or gastric mucosa were observed. The authors concluded that Stretta delivery to the gastric cardia in dogs prevents the triggering of tLESRs, thereby reducing gastroesophageal reflux.

Arts and colleagues[33] tested the hypothesis that Stretta alters GEJ resistance in a double-blind randomized crossover study of Stretta and sham treatment in patients with GERD. Twenty-two patients participated in the study, 11 in the Stretta and 11 in the sham treatment groups. Patients underwent two upper gastrointestinal endoscopies with 3 months interval, during which active or sham Stretta treatment was performed in a randomized double-blind manner. Symptom assessment, endoscopy, manometry, 24-hour esophageal pH monitoring, and a distensibility test of the GEJ using a Barostat were done before the start of the study and after 3 months. Barostat distensibility test of the GEJ before and after administration of sildenafil, an esophageal smooth muscle relaxant, was the main outcome measure. Initial sham treatment did not affect any of the parameters studied. Three months after the initial Stretta procedure, no changes were observed in esophageal acid exposure and LES pressure. In contrast, symptom score was significantly improved and GEJ compliance was significantly decreased. Administration of sildenafil normalized GEJ compliance again to pre-Stretta level, arguing against GEJ fibrosis as the underlying mechanism. The authors concluded that decreased GEJ compliance, which reflects altered LES neuromuscular function, may contribute to symptomatic benefit by decreasing refluxate volume.

STRETTA SAFETY

The Stretta procedure is safe and well-tolerated. To date, more than 25,000 Stretta procedures have been performed globally.[20] The most common complications reported have been gastroparesis and ulcerative esophagitis, which are rare. Transient epigastric pain or chest pain, low-grade fever, dysphagia, and odynophagia have also been reported.[20,34] Liu and colleagues[11] in their study involving 90 patients report five cases of dyspepsia, nine transient chest pain, two superficial mucosal injury, three mucosal bleeding, and two low-grade fever after the procedure. Rare serious complications have been described, such as esophageal perforation in three patients and two deaths caused by aspiration pneumonia.[35] The perforations were attributed to either poor patient selection or operation error. All serious adverse events occurred before 2002 and since that time there have been changes to the protocol and equipment, with no further serious adverse events reported to the Food and Drug Administration.

SUMMARY

It is the authors' opinion that the Stretta procedure is safe, well-tolerated, and produces long-lasting effects in an appropriately selected patient. In our experience, optimal candidates for Stretta seem to be patients with hiatal hernia or diaphragmatic hiatus less than 2 cm, patients with typical GERD symptoms who are partially responsive to PPI therapy, and who are predominantly upright refluxers. It is thought that the Stretta procedure increases gastric yield pressure, prevents the triggering of tLESRs, and decreases GEJ compliance. The Stretta procedure can be repeated and does not preclude any alternative intervention, such as PPI addition, further endoscopic therapy, or antireflux surgery. Novel applications for Stretta are emerging including patients who have undergone prior fundoplication or sleeve gastrectomy; however, studies in these areas are still limited.

REFERENCES

1. Peery AF, Dellon ES, Lund J, et al. Burden of gastrointestinal disease in the United States: 2012 update. Gastroenterology 2012;143(5):1179–87.e3.
2. Howell MD, Novack V, Grgurich P, et al. Iatrogenic gastric acid suppression and the risk of nosocomial *Clostridium difficile* infection. Arch Intern Med 2010;170(9): 784–90.
3. Linsky A, Gupta K, Lawler EV, et al. Proton pump inhibitors and risk for recurrent *Clostridium difficile* infection. Arch Intern Med 2010;170(9):772–8.
4. Moayyedi P, Leontiadis GI. The risks of PPI therapy. Nat Rev Gastroenterol Hepatol 2012;9(3):132–9.
5. Kahrilas PJ. Clinical practice. Gastroesophageal reflux disease. N Engl J Med 2008;359(16):1700–7.
6. Sifrim D, Zerbib F. Diagnosis and management of patients with reflux symptoms refractory to proton pump inhibitors. Gut 2012;61(9):1340–54.
7. Dean BB, Gano AD Jr, Knight K, et al. Effectiveness of proton pump inhibitors in nonerosive reflux disease. Clin Gastroenterol Hepatol 2004;2(8):656–64.
8. Kahrilas PJ, Boeckxstaens G. Failure of reflux inhibitors in clinical trials: bad drugs or wrong patients? Gut 2012;61(10):1501–9.
9. Lagergren J, Bergstrom R, Lindgren A, et al. Symptomatic gastroesophageal reflux as a risk factor for esophageal adenocarcinoma. N Engl J Med 1999;340(11): 825–31.
10. Finks JF, Wei Y, Birkmeyer JD. The rise and fall of antireflux surgery in the United States. Surg Endosc 2006;20(11):1698–701.
11. Liu HF, Zhang JG, Li J, et al. Improvement of clinical parameters in patients with gastroesophageal reflux disease after radiofrequency energy delivery. World J Gastroenterol 2011;17(39):4429–33.
12. Triadafilopoulos G, DiBaise JK, Nostrant TT, et al. The Stretta procedure for the treatment of GERD: 6 and 12 month follow-up of the U.S. open label trial. Gastrointest Endosc 2002;55(2):149–56.

13. Corley DA, Katz P, Wo JM, et al. Improvement of gastroesophageal reflux symptoms after radiofrequency energy: a randomized, sham-controlled trial. Gastroenterology 2003;125(3):668–76.
14. Coron E, Sebille V, Cadiot G, et al. Clinical trial: radiofrequency energy delivery in proton pump inhibitor-dependent gastro-oesophageal reflux disease patients. Aliment Pharmacol Ther 2008;28(9):1147–58.
15. Dughera L, Navino M, Cassolino P, et al. Long-term results of radiofrequency energy delivery for the treatment of GERD: results of a prospective 48-month study. Diagn Ther Endosc 2011;2011:507157.
16. Noar MD, Lotfi-Emran S. Sustained improvement in symptoms of GERD and antisecretory drug use: 4-year follow-up of the Stretta procedure. Gastrointest Endosc 2007;65(3):367–72.
17. Reymunde A, Santiago N. Long-term results of radiofrequency energy delivery for the treatment of GERD: sustained improvements in symptoms, quality of life, and drug use at 4-year follow-up. Gastrointest Endosc 2007;65(3):361–6.
18. Dughera L, Rotondano G, De Cento M, et al. Durability of Stretta radiofrequency treatment for GERD: results of an 8-year follow-up. Gastroenterol Res Pract 2014; 2014:531907.
19. Noar M, Squires P, Noar E, et al. Long-term maintenance effect of radiofrequency energy delivery for refractory GERD: a decade later. Surg Endosc 2014;28(8): 2323–33.
20. Perry KA, Banerjee A, Melvin WS. Radiofrequency energy delivery to the lower esophageal sphincter reduces esophageal acid exposure and improves GERD symptoms: a systematic review and meta-analysis. Surg Laparosc Endosc Percutan Tech 2012;22(4):283–8.
21. Milkes D, Gerson LB, Triadafilopoulos G. Complete elimination of reflux symptoms does not guarantee normalization of intraesophageal and intragastric pH in patients with gastroesophageal reflux disease (GERD). Am J Gastroenterol 2004;99(6):991–6.
22. Aziz AM, El-Khayat HR, Sadek A, et al. A prospective randomized trial of sham, single-dose Stretta, and double-dose Stretta for the treatment of gastroesophageal reflux disease. Surg Endosc 2010;24(4):818–25.
23. Dundon JM, Davis SS, Hazey JW, et al. Radiofrequency energy delivery to the lower esophageal sphincter (Stretta procedure) does not provide long-term symptom control. Surg Innov 2008;15(4):297–301.
24. Lipka S, Kumar A, Richter JE. No evidence for efficacy of radiofrequency ablation for treatment of gastroesophageal reflux disease: a systematic review and meta-analysis. Clin Gastroenterol Hepatol 2015;13(6):1058–10567.e1.
25. Fass R, Cahn F, Scotti DJ, et al. Systematic review and meta-analysis of controlled and prospective cohort efficacy studies of endoscopic radiofrequency for treatment of gastroesophageal reflux disease. Surg Endosc 2017;31(12): 4865–82.
26. Khidir N, Angrisani L, Al-Qahtani J, et al. Initial experience of endoscopic radiofrequency waves delivery to the lower esophageal sphincter (Stretta Procedure) on symptomatic gastroesophageal reflux disease post-sleeve gastrectomy. Obes Surg 2018;28(10):3125–30.
27. Noar M, Squires P, Khan S. Radiofrequency energy delivery to the lower esophageal sphincter improves gastroesophageal reflux patient-reported outcomes in failed laparoscopic Nissen fundoplication cohort. Surg Endosc 2017;31(7): 2854–62.

28. Fry LC, Monkemuller K, Malfertheiner P. Systematic review: endoluminal therapy for gastro-oesophageal reflux disease: evidence from clinical trials. Eur J Gastroenterol Hepatol 2007;19(12):1125–39.
29. Triadafilopoulos G. Stretta: an effective, minimally invasive treatment for gastroesophageal reflux disease. Am J Med 2003;115(Suppl 3A):192S–200S.
30. Triadafilopoulos G. Stretta: a valuable endoscopic treatment modality for gastroesophageal reflux disease. World J Gastroenterol 2014;20(24):7730–8.
31. Utley DS, Kim M, Vierra MA, et al. Augmentation of lower esophageal sphincter pressure and gastric yield pressure after radiofrequency energy delivery to the gastroesophageal junction: a porcine model. Gastrointest Endosc 2000; 52(1):81–6.
32. Kim MS, Holloway RH, Dent J, et al. Radiofrequency energy delivery to the gastric cardia inhibits triggering of transient lower esophageal sphincter relaxation and gastroesophageal reflux in dogs. Gastrointest Endosc 2003;57(1):17–22.
33. Arts J, Bisschops R, Blondeau K, et al. A double-blind sham-controlled study of the effect of radiofrequency energy on symptoms and distensibility of the gastroesophageal junction in GERD. Am J Gastroenterol 2012;107(2):222–30.
34. Chen D, Barber C, McLoughlin P, et al. Systematic review of endoscopic treatments for gastro-oesophageal reflux disease. Br J Surg 2009;96(2):128–36.
35. Gersin K, Fanelli R. The Stretta procedure: review of catheter and technique evolution. Surg Endosc 2002;16:PF199.

Transoral Incisionless Fundoplication

Kenneth J. Chang, MD, FASGE, FACG, AGAF, FJGES[a],*, Reginald Bell, MD, FACS[b]

KEYWORDS

- Esophagitis • Fundoplication • Gastroesophageal reflux • Hiatal hernia • Humans
- Laparoscopy • Proton pump inhibitors • Treatment outcome reflux

KEY POINTS

- On the GERD spectrum, TIF may be a treatment option among patients with GERD with an intact and functioning crura, but would benefit from strengthening, tightening, and lengthening the LES complex. Therefore, patient selection is very important in determining which patients will likely have the best outcome.
- As an endoscopic procedure, TIF reduces EGJ distensibility, thereby decreasing tLESRs, and also creates a 3-cm high-pressure zone at the distal esophagus in the configuration of a flap valve.
- Level 1 evidence confirms both the safety and efficacy of TIF 2.0, especially in patients who have troublesome regurgitation despite PPI therapy.
- The concomitant laparoscopic hernia repair with TIF for those patients with hiatal hernia greater than 2 cm is now emerging as a potential strategy within laparoscopic antireflux surgery.
- Future potential applications that are currently being investigated include the use of TIF in (1) patients with Barrett's esophagus; (2) patients with achalasia after per-oral endoscopic myotomy; (3) bariatric patients before and after laparoscopic sleeve gastrectomy; and (4) patients after lung transplant.

INTRODUCTION

Gastroesophageal reflux disease (GERD) results from an incompetent barrier resisting the retrograde movement of gastric content. This mechanical defect can be restored with various techniques, one of which involves advancing and fixing the gastric fundus around the lower esophagus using a transoral longitudinal and rotational technique. The purpose of this article is to review the rationale, mechanisms of action,

Author contributions: K.J. Chang and R. Bell designed the overall concept, the outline of the article, and were responsible for writing and editing of the article.

[a] Gastroenterology and Hepatology Division, H.H. Chao Comprehensive Digestive Disease Center, University of California, Irvine Medical Center, 101 The City Drive, Orange, CA 92868, USA; [b] Institute of Esophageal and Reflux Surgery, 499 East Hampden Avenue #400, Englewood, CO 80113, USA

* Corresponding author.

E-mail address: kchang@uci.edu

https://doi.org/10.1016/j.giec.2019.12.008
1052-5157/20/© 2020 Elsevier Inc. All rights reserved.
giendo.theclinics.com

appropriate patient selection, technical aspects, clinical results, safety, and emerging application of the procedure known as transoral incisionless fundoplication (TIF 2.0).

WHY TRANSORAL INCISIONLESS FUNDOPLICATION?

GERD is the most prevalent gastrointestinal disorder in the United States,[1] and the extent of anatomic alterations underlying the mechanism of GERD can be viewed as a spectrum from normal to a single anatomic alteration (eg, weak lower esophageal sphincter [LES]) to multiple anatomic alterations, such as weak LES, open diaphragmatic hiatus, and hiatal hernia (**Fig. 1**).[2,3] The degree of anatomic alterations also seem to correlate with the complications of GERD, namely degree of esophagitis, the presence of Barrett's metaplasia[4] dysplasia and its progression to esophageal adenocarcinoma. Thus, as GERD is a spectrum disorder, treatment should be individualized to the anatomic alterations of each patient. Although medical and surgical therapy have been the mainstay of treatment of GERD, there are currently several Food and Drug Administration (FDA)-approved devices available for endoscopic treatment of GERD, thus filling the therapeutic gap between medications and surgery. Endoscopic treatment options are now considered appropriate treatment in patients early in the GERD spectrum.

HOW DOES IT WORK?

Pressure gradients between the abdominal stomach and thoracic esophagus would favor retrograde movement of gastric contents into the esophagus during much of human activity, were it not for a complex antireflux mechanism at the juncture of the esophagus, stomach, and diaphragm. One of the 2 primary components to this antireflux barrier is intrinsic to the esophagus and comprises the LES and esophagogastric junction (EGJ). The second component is the crural diaphragm, which in a normal individual acts in concert with the LES to open during swallowing and then contract, pinching the esophagus, to maximize the threshold preventing gastric reflux. The 2 components taken together constitute the high-pressure zone (HPZ) found during esophageal manometry, and high-resolution manometry demonstrates that both the crural diaphragm and the LES open synchronously during swallowing and belching.

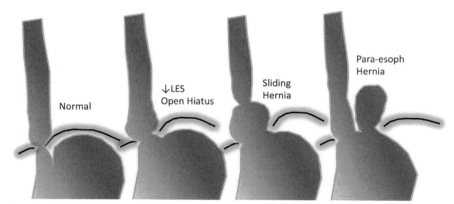

Fig. 1. Spectrum of anatomic defects among patients with gastroesophageal reflux disease. LES, lower esophageal sphincter.

Transient or permanent mechanical dysfunction of one or both of these components is a prerequisite for GERD. In early stages of GERD, transient opening of the HPZ occurs too frequently and is too often accompanied by reflux of gastric contents rather than merely air. Whether this occurs because of a neurologic reflex or transient shortening of the LES leading to loss of sphincteric competence has been a topic of debate; regardless, antireflux procedures, such as Nissen fundoplication have been found to decrease both the frequency of these transient events as well as the amount of gastric liquid reflux during these transient events. In more advanced stages of GERD, a chronic loss of LES length and pressure, and separation of crural diaphragm from the LES due to hiatal hernia, lead to more severe reflux.

Even though acid-reducing medication is the mainstay of treating GERD, medication does not decrease the frequency of reflux events, and persistent symptoms related to ongoing reflux often require a mechanical solution. Historically open or laparoscopic fundoplication procedures have been considered the "gold standard" intervention to restore the antireflux barrier because they enable restoration of both the crural component by hiatal hernia repair and the LES by creating a flap valve via fundoplication. However, both the level of invasiveness, and the gas-bloat side effects related to a supracompetent flap valve, have led to a search for alternative interventions.

In patients who have a largely intact crural sphincter (ie, absence or a very limited hiatal hernia, Hill grade 1 or 2), the potential for an endoluminal approach to restoring the LES exists. Conceptually this could entail decreasing the distensibility of the whole or just the bottom of the LES to prevent shortening and loss of LES competence during gastric distention, increasing the resting pressure of the LES, reinforcing the sling fibers at the gastroesophageal (GE) junction (**Fig. 2**), or locally altering vagal neuromodulation of transient LES openings.

Although early attempts at endoscopic fundoplication were unsuccessful and lacked durability, more robust devices and techniques designed to physically reconstruct a flap valve, namely the TIF procedure, have resulted in more successful and durable restoration of LES function, and have done so without the degree of side effects seen with a Nissen fundoplication. In its current technique iteration (TIF 2.0), this procedure is anatomically and physiologically similar to surgical fundoplication (**Fig. 3**). During the procedure, the gastric fundus is folded up and around the distal esophagus, which has been retracted below the diaphragm, and anchored with polypropylene fasteners. This results in tightening and reinforcing the sling fibers (see **Fig. 2**A, B) of the proximal stomach (the lower portion of the LES), accentuating the cardiac notch, steepening the angle of His, and reestablishing the flap valve mechanism. One can argue that, although both Nissen and TIF create a HPZ at the GE junction,[5] the TIF 2.0 procedure is actually creating a true flap valve.

The mechanism of action of the TIF procedure in many ways mirrors that of the Nissen laparoscopic antireflux surgery (LARS).[5] One paper, published by Rinsma and colleagues[6] characterizes such mechanisms. In their study involving 15 patients, they performed 90-minute postprandial combined with high-resolution manometry and impedance-pH monitoring followed by an ambulatory 24-hour pH-impedance monitoring. EGJ distensibility was evaluated using an endoscopic functional luminal imaging probe before and directly after the procedures. The patients were followed for 6 months. With regard to the stationary esophageal manometry and impedance-pH monitoring performed directly after the procedure, TIF 2.0 resulted in a marked reduction of both the number of transient LES relaxation episodes (tLESRs) (16.8 ± 1.5 versus 9.2 ± 1.3; $P<.01$) and the number of tLESRs associated with liquid-containing reflux after the procedure (from 11.1 ± 1.6 versus 5.6 ± 0.6; $P<.01$). TIF

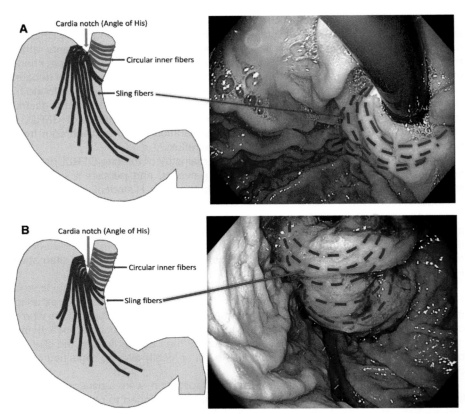

Fig. 2. Diagram and image of the muscle fibers in the distal esophagus (circular inner fibers) and proximal stomach (sling fibers) that make up the entirety of the lower esophageal sphincter. (*A*) Pre-TIF valve showing "flat" angle of His (Cardia Notch), short valve, and loose gastric sling fibers. (*B*) Post-TIF valve showing "steep" angle of His (Cardia Notch), tall valve, and tighter gastric sling fibers.

Principles Of Antireflux Surgery	TIF 2.0 Procedure	Laparoscopic Fundoplication
Reduce hiatal hernia ≤2 cm	✓	✓
Repair hiatal hernia >2 cm and close crura	✓ [a]	✓
Elongate the intraabdominal esophagus	✓	✓
Fundoplication	✓	✓
• Approximate and tighten the fundus around the distal esophagus	✓	✓
• Recreate the dynamics of the angle of His	✓	✓
• Restore the distal high pressure zone	✓	✓

Fig. 3. Applying the Principles of Antireflux Surgery to Laparoscopic Fundoplication and TIF 2.0. All of the principal elements are preserved in both. [a] As of June 22, 2017, EsophyX device indication was expanded to include patients with hiatal hernias larger than 2 cm, where a laparoscopic hiatal hernia repair (HHR) reduces the hernia to 2 cm or less. (*Courtesy of* EndoGastric Solutions, Redmond, WA; with permission.)

also led to a decrease in the number and proximal extent of reflux episodes and an improvement of acid exposure in the upright position; conversely, TIF had no effect on the number of gas reflux episodes, corroborating the low incidence of post-TIF gas-bloat symptoms. EGJ distensibility was reduced after the procedure (2.4 ± 0.3 versus 1.6 ± 0.2 mm^2/mm Hg; $P<.05$). Also of note, the basal LES pressure in the fasted state was increased after TIF (from 13.9 ± 1.0 to 20.5 ± 1.8 mm Hg; $P<.01$). Thus, TIF reduces EGJ distensibility, thereby decreasing tLESRs, which is the main mechanism for upright refluxers. It also creates a 3-cm HPZ at the distal esophagus in the configuration of a flap valve, which should decrease both upright and supine reflux. However, because it is a 270° partial fundoplication, and the flap valve luminal diameter is controlled by the diameter of the device (preventing over-tightening), gas can still escape from the stomach into the esophagus, minimizing the gas-bloat side effect.

WHICH PATIENTS SHOULD CONSIDER TIF?

Patient selection for TIF is critical. First, the patient must have a clear indication for an antireflux procedure (see Rena Yadlapati and John E. Pandolfino's article, "Personalized Approach in the Work-up and Management of GERD," in this issue). One must then discern which patients are good candidates for TIF alone, and which patients are better served with a laparoscopic or combined approach (see the Concomitant Laparoscopic Hernia Repair and Transoral Incisionless Fundoplication section, below). We like to discuss with our patients that there are actually 2 "valves" that prevent reflux: the "inside valve" (LES) and the "outside valve" (crura). In addition, there are 3 components of the antireflux anatomy that we need to assess: (1) whether there is a hiatal hernia that needs to be reduced, (2) whether the right crura, which acts like a sling or noose around the GE junction[7,8] (see Robin A. Zachariah and colleagues' article, "Mechanism and Pathophysiology of GERD," in this issue), needs to be tightened, and (3) whether the LES needs to have a valve reconstruction. The axial or vertical length of the hiatal hernia can be assessed by an esophagram or upper endoscopy. Neither modality is perfect, as sliding hernias can often be missed. Even more tricky, however, is the assessment of the crural tightness (diaphragmatic hiatus). The Hill classification performed during a retroflex view is the most effective way to quantify the crural opening. However, this can often be misleading (ie, underestimating the Hill grade) for the following reasons: (1) insufficient time and insufflation during retroflex (**Fig. 4**) and (2) a fat pad can fill the open hiatus, creating a "stuffing" affect (**Fig. 5**). We recommend 60 seconds be spent in retroflex with active insufflation to determine the Hill classification. A Hill grade 1 or 2 is acceptable for TIF alone. However, if the hiatus is open more than 2 cm (or 2 scope diameters, ie, Hill 3), or there is an axial hernia length of more than 2 cm (Hill 4), the patient will most likely need a crural repair, which cannot be accomplished with TIF alone. We call this the 2 × 2 rule. In our experience, underestimation of the Hill grade is the most common reason for TIF failure. This cannot be overemphasized. In a paper describing salvage laparoscopic surgery among 5 patients who failed TIF, 3 of the 5 patients were found to have significant hiatal hernia that required repair at the time of revision.[9]

HOW DO WE DO IT?

The TIF 2.0 procedure is performed using the disposable, single-use, EsophyX Z+ device (EndoGastric Solutions, Redmond, WA), designed to create full-thickness serosa-to-serosa plications and reconstruct valves approximately 3 cm in length, and 200° to 300° in circumference (**Fig. 6**). The device is comprised of an 18-mm-diameter frame

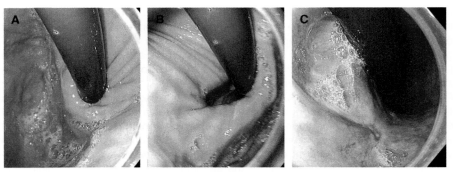

Fig. 4. The "60 seconds rule" for assessing the diaphragmatic hiatus in retroflexed position underscores the common mistake of underestimating the Hill grade. (*A*) Initially, after only a few seconds of inspection, assessment appears to be a Hill grade 1. (*B*) About 30 seconds later, with continuous CO_2 insufflation and scope rotation, the hiatus opens up to Hill grade 2, approximately 2 cm in diameter. (*C*) At close to 60 seconds, the hiatus opens even wider to approximately 3 cm in diameter.

through which a standard endoscope can be introduced (**Fig. 7**A); a handle with controls; tissue invaginator (**Fig. 7**B), consisting of side holes positioned at the distal end of the frame to which external suction can be applied; the tissue mold (**Fig. 7**C), which pushes tissue against the chassis of the device; a helical retractor (**Fig. 7**D), which is advanced into the tissue and allows for the retraction of the tissue between the tissue mold and the chassis; 2 stylets (**Fig. 7**E) that puncture the plicated tissue and tissue mold, and over which polypropylene H-shaped fasteners can be deployed; and a cartridge (**Fig. 7**F) that holds 20 fasteners.

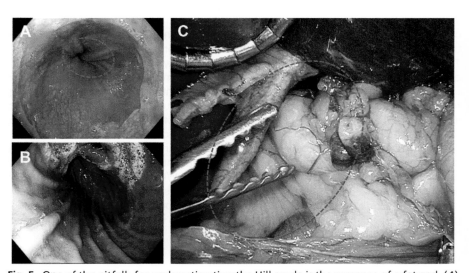

Fig. 5. One of the pitfalls for underestimating the Hill grade is the presence of a fat pad. (*A*) Antegrade view of the GE junction (*blue circle*) seems to be normal. (*B*) Retroflex view appears to be a Hill grade 2. (*C*) Concomitant laparoscopic view showing a 3 × 2-cm open hiatus that is "stuffed" with fat, which compresses the GE junction resulting in underestimation of an actual Hill grade 3 anatomy by endoscopy.

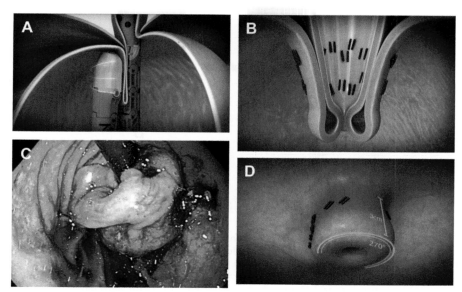

Fig. 6. The goal of TIF 2.0 is to create full-thickness serosa-to-serosa plications with the reconstruction of a valve that is 200° to 300° in circumference and 3 cm in length. (*A*) Traction of tissue into the EsophyX Z+ device results in the full 3-cm length neo valve reconstruction. (*B*) Full-thickness serosa-to-serosa plications cause fibroelastic tissue deposition and tissue adhesion for a durable valve. (*C*) The end results is a GE junction that is narrower, longer, and floppy. (*D*) Endoscopic image immediately after TIF showing a 4-cm length valve that is nearly circumferential. (*Courtesy of* EndoGastric Solutions, Redmond, WA; with permission.)

We perform the procedure under general anesthesia with muscle relaxation and positive pressure ventilation to aid in reducing any hernia, in the supine position to decrease pressure on the GE junction from the liver. Before the start of the procedure, it is helpful to first perform a diagnostic esophagogastroduodenoscopy examination to measure the length from the patient's incisors to the Z-line as well as the diaphragmatic pinch, note any anatomic abnormalities, and verify that the stomach is free of food contents. If there is any question about the compatibility of the endoscope, the Endoscopy Compatibility Tool can be used to verify that the diameter of the endoscope will be compatible with the EsophyX Z+.

The endoscope is then liberally coated with lubricant, and lubricant is also placed over the endoscope seal of the EsophyX Z+ device. The endoscope is then inserted through the seal and advanced until the endoscope tip extends approximately 10 to 15 cm beyond the distal tip of the device. Lubricant is then reapplied over the distal end of the endoscope and the distal two-thirds of the device. Predilation using an over-the-wire dilator (54 or 57 Fr) may be used to relax the hypopharynx and upper esophageal sphincter. The device is then placed in the patient's oral cavity, gently advanced under direct visualization, and advanced into the stomach. The device tissue mold will occasionally encounter resistance as it passes through the larynx and cricopharyngeus, and jaw thrust may aid safe passage. Sometimes having the anesthesiologist deflate the balloon of the endotracheal tube for just a few minutes will also help the device to pass through the hypopharynx. The stomach is insufflated (using an autoregulated CO_2 insufflator

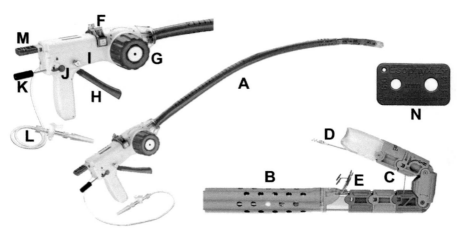

Fig. 7. The multiple parts and features of the EsophyX Z+ device. (A) Flexible shaft with measurement markings. (B) Invaginator suction ports that "couple" the device shaft to the tubular esophagus to aid in reducing a small hernia and in "pushing off the diaphragm." (C) Tissue mold that opens and closes to capture and rotate tissue for plication. (D) Helical retractor to retract tissue into the tissue mold to create valve length. (E) Stylets with H-shaped fasteners are "fired" from the shaft, through tissue, and into the receiving clear plastic chamber at the distal tip of the device. (F) Fastener cartridge containing 20 polypropylene fasteners that load 2 at a time. (G) Tissue mold knob that opens and closes the tissue mold. It has a ratchet mechanism that precludes backwards slippage of the wheel and a safety feature that precludes overtightening. (H) Fastener delivery trigger, which fires the stylets and fasteners across the tissue mold. (I) Fastener delivery trigger release, which must be depressed to release the trigger handle. (J) Helical retractor control lock, which, once in lock position, still allows the retractor to be pulled back, but does not allow slippage away from the device. (K) Helical retractor control, clockwise rotation of which allows insertion into tissue and counter-clockwise rotation to come off tissue. (L) Stop cock for invaginator, which connects suction to the invaginator ports. (M) Fastener pushers, which receive and push the fasteners down to the distal end of the device. (N) Endoscope compatibility tool, used to confirm that the endoscope will fit into the device. (*Courtesy of* EndoGastric Solutions, Redmond, WA; with permission.)

set to 15–18 mm Hg) through the working channel of the flexible endoscope, and the endoscope is positioned in retroflexion. Under direct visualization, the device is further advanced into the stomach until the second blue segment is seen entering the stomach, and then rotated to align the back of the tissue mold to the lesser curve of the stomach. The endoscope is retracted into the distal aspect of the chassis, and the tissue mold is closed. The endoscope is then re-advanced into the stomach through the side hole and placed back in retroflexion to visualize the EsophyX Z+ device and the GE junction (**Fig. 8**).

If there is a small hiatal hernia, the device can be withdrawn back into the distal esophagus, where suction is applied to engage the distal esophageal mucosa. The device can then be advanced to bring the herniated stomach back below the diaphragm.

Using the positions on a clock face, with 12 o'clock precisely on the lesser curve (**Fig. 9**), we usually begin at the posterior corner, which is toward the 11 o'clock position. If possible, we try to plant the helical retractor as close to 12 o'clock as possible (for both posterior and anterior corners), which allows for maximal folding of the fundus around the esophagus (**Fig. 10**); this has become known as the "Bell Roll."[10]

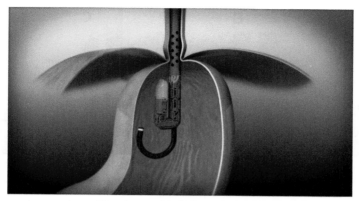

Fig. 8. The endoscope in position to provide light and visualization of the working end of the EsophyX Z+ device. The scope is first withdrawn from the distal tip back into the channel, the tissue mold is then closed, and the scope is re-advanced through the side port to assume this position. (*Courtesy of* EndoGastric Solutions, Redmond, WA; with permission.)

The helical retractor is now advanced until it is in contact with tissue just below the squamocolumnar junction, and the helical retractor control is rotated clockwise to engage tissue (**Fig. 11**). The mold and retractor are advanced by 1 cm, and the mold is opened slightly to release the retractor from the tissue mold. The entire device

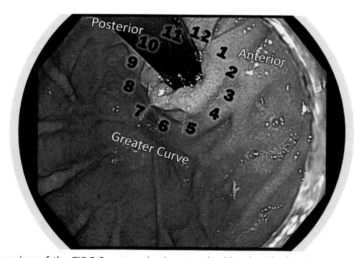

Fig. 9. Mapping of the TIF 2.0 protocol using standard landmarks for placement of the helical retractor and rotation toward the lesser curve. Using the positions on a clock face, with 12 o'clock precisely on the lesser curve we usually begin at the posterior corner, placing the retractor as close to 12 o'clock as possible, and rotating the tissue clockwise toward the lesser curve. After 3 plications in the posterior side, the device is rotated to the anterior side and 3 additional plications are placed with counter-clockwise wrapping of the fundus toward the lesser curve. Then the helix is secured at 5 o'clock and 2 plications are placed here (5 and 6 o'clock). The helix is then secured at 7 o'clock and 2 additional plications are placed here (7 and 8 o'clock). These last 4 plications on the greater curve do not involve any tissue rotation/wrapping.

A   B   C

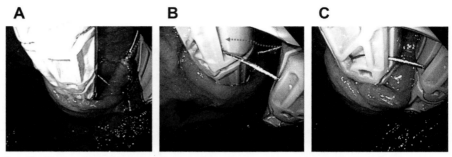

Fig. 10. The "Bell Roll" technique on the anterior corner. (*A*) With the helical retractor firmly secured at 12 o'clock, (*B*) the tissue mold is rotated back out to 6 o'clock, followed by de-sufflation and retraction of tissue; then (*C*) the tissue mold is rotated back toward the lesser curve, capturing the fundic tissue and wrapping it toward the back of the esophagus.

is then withdrawn to a level such that the proximal blue segment is above the GE junction (**Fig. 12**). This "sets" the device so that the 2 sharp stylets will exit the device approximately 1.5 cm proximal to blue segment.

While desufflating, the retractor is pulled down maximally (this excursion length will determine the length of the neo valve) (**Fig. 13**). With retraction, this tissue is pulled in between the tissue mold and the chassis. Once fully retracted (around 3 cm), rotation toward the lesser curve is started using a counter-clockwise motion with the handle. This will result in a clockwise rotation on the monitor. It is a combination of retraction and rotation that will optimize the wrap.

Once retraction and rotation is complete, there is a stepwise sequence that ensues, which is likened to a little "dance" called "lock, lock, suck; push off the diaphragm; fire" (**Fig. 14**). The first "lock" is to lock the helical retractor (see **Fig. 7**J). The second "lock" is to close and lock the tissue mold (see **Fig. 7**G). The "suck" is to have the assistant turn on the invaginator suction (see **Fig. 7**L) to couple the esophagus with the device (analogous to tight jeans or a wet suit, see **Fig. 14**B, C). At this point the

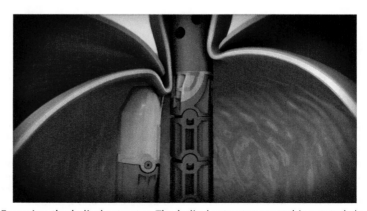

Fig. 11. Engaging the helical retractor. The helical retractor control is rotated clockwise to engage tissue, ideally right at the squamocolumnar junction where it tends to be most secure. (*Courtesy of* EndoGastric Solutions, Redmond, WA; with permission.)

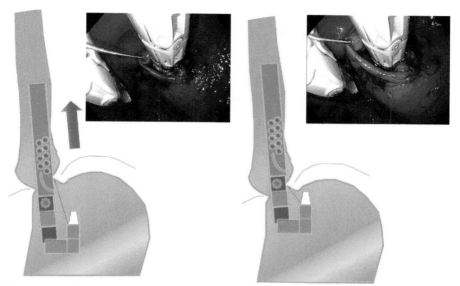

Fig. 12. "Set" the device. The entire device is then withdrawn to a level such that the proximal blue segment is above the GE junction. This "sets" the device so that the 2 sharp stylets will exit the device approximately 1.5 cm proximal to blue segment.

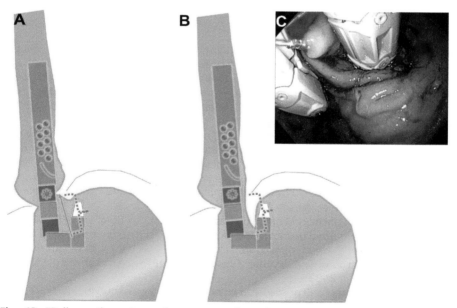

Fig. 13. "Pull on the retractor" to create the valve length. (*A*) While desufflating, the retractor is pulled down maximally (this excursion length will determine the length of the neo valve). (*B*) With retraction, this tissue is pulled in between the tissue mold and the chassis. (*C*) Once fully retracted (around 3 cm length, the helix wire is maximally shorten), begin rotation toward the lesser curve using a counter-clockwise motion with the handle. This will result in a clockwise rotation on the monitor. It is a combination of retraction and rotation that will optimize the wrap.

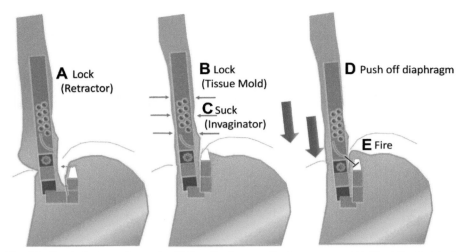

Fig. 14. "Lock, lock, suck, push off the diaphragm, fire" sequence. (A) "Lock"—first lock the helical retractor control lock. (B) "Lock"—then lock the tissue mold. (C) "Suck"—turn on the stop cock to apply suction to the invaginator ports. (D) "Push off the diaphragm"—with the device and esophagus now coupled via suction, push the device 0.5 to 1.0 cm distally to ensure that the stylet and fasteners do not penetrate through the diaphragm, but fire below the diaphragm. (E) "Fire"—depress the fastener delivery trigger release followed by squeezing the fastener delivery trigger. After this, one should reload the fasteners, release the suction, reinsufflate, and repeat as necessary.

stomach is reinsufflated. "Push off the diaphragm" means that the scope and device (as one construct) are re-advanced to the initial length of the GE junction (see **Fig. 14**D), which ensures that the stylets do not fire into and through the diaphragm muscles. Fasteners are loaded (if not done already), and finally "fire" (see **Fig. 14**E) by depressing the safety button (see **Fig. 7**I) and squeezing the trigger (see **Fig. 7**H) to deploy the double fasteners (see **Fig. 7**E).

At this time, the fasteners can be reloaded, and the invaginator turned off. The device is rotated out of the corner, and the retractor is unlocked and the tissue mold opened. This sequence is repeated for the second and third plications into the posterior corner. After 3 plications, the tissue mold is opened and the helical retractor removed. The device is then rotated to the anterior corner (**Fig. 15**), and an additional 3 plications are performed here.

Then, the device is positioned at the 5 o'clock and 7 o'clock positions (**Fig. 16**A–C). Here the main goal is retraction (no rotation at these positions) to gain additional length at the greater curve. These steps are repeated, taking 2 plications with the retractor at 5 o'clock (plicate at 5, 6) and another 2 plications with the retractor relocated to 7 o'clock (plicate at 7 and 8 o'clock).

After these 10 plications (3 posterior, 3 anterior, and 4 greater curve), which result in 20 fasteners deployed, whether further plications are necessary must be assessed. Typically, an additional 2 to 8 bites are performed to visual satisfaction (see **Fig. 16**D). As one becomes more proficient with the standard technique described here, there is room for "tailoring" the plications to the individual's anatomy. For example, in patients with previous failed Nissen fundoplication, one needs to consider where the previous fundoplication is intact and the areas of opportunity for TIF revision.

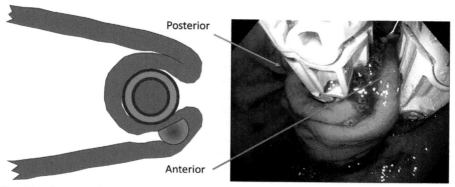

Fig. 15. After completing 3 plications in the posterior corner, the device is rotated to the anterior corner. The same sequences shown in **Figs. 11–14** are now repeated in the anterior corner.

HOW WELL DOES IT WORK?

The TIF technique has undergone significant evolution from a gastrogastric plication to an esophagogastric plication, with various degrees of roll and depth. In addition

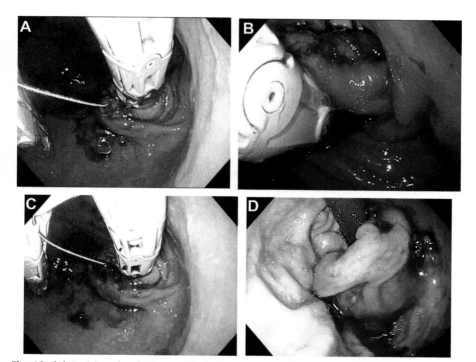

Fig. 16. (A) Position the device and helical retractor at the 5 o'clock and (C) 7 o'clock positions. (B) While desufflating, the retractor is pulled down maximally, (here there is no rotation into the corners), followed by same steps as in Figure 14. Here the main goal is retraction to gain additional length at the greater curve. Repeat these steps, taking 2 plications with the retractor at 5 o'clock (plicate at 5, 6) and another 2 plications with the retractor relocated to 7 o'clock (plicate at 7 and 8'oclock). (D) Completed Valve.

to technique modifications, the device itself has undergone several major iterations to improve ease of use, improve fastener delivery, and enable fastener delivery without having to visualize the stylet/fastener deployment. With improved ease of use, the proceduralist has been able to focus more on a standardized technique. With the ability to deploy fasteners without visualizing deployment enables a greater degree of rotational movement, which, at least on the anterior aspect of the fundoplication, can be significant. These enhancements have led to significantly better reproducibility and outcomes than the previous versions of EsophyX.

An additional aspect of evaluating outcomes concerns the relation of classic study design to patient-centric care. For most study designs, continued proton pump inhibitor (PPI) use in some form has been used as a measure of failure. However, most patients coming to antireflux interventions are not adequately controlled on medication (hence the decision to have an invasive procedure). A patient-centric approach would argue that a successful intervention would include taking a patient with persistent, uncontrolled symptoms on medication, to having controlled symptoms regardless of medication use.

There have been more than a dozen noncomparative studies evaluating the most current TIF 2.0 procedure.[11–22] There have also been multiple analyses of published studies, and rather than repeat the same we will highlight the level 1 data here.

There have been 3 recent randomized control clinical trials using TIF 2.0, which uses the most advanced technique, similar to LARS. The first, known as the TEMPO trial, consisted of 63 patients randomized to TIF (40 patients) versus high-dose PPI (23 patients).[23] The primary outcome was elimination of daily troublesome regurgitation or extraesophageal symptoms. Secondary outcomes were normalization of esophageal acid exposure, PPI use, and healing of esophagitis. At the 6-month follow-up, troublesome regurgitation was eliminated in 97% of patients who had undergone TIF versus 50% of patients on PPIs (relative risk [RR] = 1.9; 95% CI, 1.2–3.11; P = .006). Globally, 62% of patients who had undergone TIF experienced elimination of regurgitation and extraesophageal symptoms versus 5% of patients on PPIs (RR = 12.9; CI, 1.9–88.9; P = .009). Esophageal acid exposure was normalized in 54% of patients who had undergone TIF versus 52% of patients on PPIs (RR = 1.0; 95% CI, 0.6–1.7; P = .914). A total of 90% of patients who had undergone TIF were off PPIs. The authors concluded that, at the 6-month follow-up, TIF was more effective than maximum standard dose PPI therapy in eliminating troublesome regurgitation and extraesophageal symptoms of GERD. Of the 63 patients receiving TIF, 5 year follow-up data were available as follows: 60 were available at 1 year, 52 at 3 years, and 44 at 5 years.[21] Troublesome regurgitation was eliminated in 88% of patients at 1 year, 90% at 3 years, and 86% at 5 years. Resolution of troublesome atypical symptoms was achieved in 82% of patients at 1 year, 88% at 3 years, and 80% at 5 years. No serious adverse events occurred. There were 3 reoperations by the end of the 5-year follow-up (5%). At the 5-year follow-up, 34% of patients were on daily PPI therapy as compared with 100% of patients at screening. The total GERD-HRQL (health-related quality of life) score improved by decreasing from 22.2 to 6.8 at 5 years (P<.001). This paper concluded that most patients undergoing TIF 2.0 experienced a durable elimination of troublesome GERD symptoms with no severe adverse events (SAEs) or safety concerns, and that TIF 2.0 could be a cost-effective alternative to laparoscopic Nissen fundoplication.

The second clinical trial studying TIF 2.0 against PPIs was the RESPECT trial,[24] which was a prospective, sham-controlled trial to determine if TIF reduced troublesome regurgitation to a greater extent than PPIs in patients with GERD. A total of 696 patients with troublesome regurgitation despite daily PPI with 3 validated

GERD-specific symptom scales, on and off PPIs, were initially screened. Of these, 87 patients with GERD and hiatal hernias ≤2 cm were randomly assigned to groups that underwent TIF and then received 6 months of placebo, or sham surgery and 6 months of once- or twice-daily omeprazole (controls, n = 42). Patients were blinded to therapy during the follow-up period and reassessed at 2, 12, and 26 weeks. At 6 months, patients underwent 48-hour esophageal pH monitoring and esophagoduodenoscopy. By intention-to-treat analysis, TIF eliminated troublesome regurgitation in a larger proportion of patients (67%) than PPIs (45%) (P = .023). A larger proportion of controls had no response at 3 months (36%) than patients who received TIF (11%) (P = .004). Control of esophageal pH improved after TIF (mean 9.3% before and 6.3% after; P<.001), but not after sham surgery (mean 8.6% before and 8.9% after). Patients from both groups who completed the protocol had similar reduction in GERD symptom scores. The authors concluded that TIF was an effective treatment for patients with GERD symptoms, particularly in those with persistent regurgitation despite PPI therapy, based on evaluation 6 months after the procedure.

The third clinical trial performed in a European study was a double-blind sham-controlled study in patients with GERD who were chronic users of PPIs.[25] Forty-four patients were randomized equally to 22 patients in each group. The primary effectiveness endpoint was the proportion of patients in clinical remission after a 6-month follow-up. Secondary outcomes were: PPI consumption, esophageal acid exposure, reduction in Quality of Life in Reflux and Dyspepsia and Gastrointestinal Symptom Rating Scale scores and healing of reflux esophagitis. Results showed that the time in remission after TIF procedure (197 days) was significantly longer compared with those submitted to the sham intervention (107 days) (P<.001). After 6 months, 13/22 (59%) of the patients with chronic GERD remained in clinical remission after TIF.

A recent meta-analysis[26] was conducted using data only from these 3 randomized studies that assessed the TIF 2.0 procedure compared with a control. The purpose of the meta-analysis was to determine the efficacy and long-term outcomes associated with performance of the TIF 2.0 procedure in patients with chronic long-term refractory GERD on optimized PPI therapy, including esophageal pH, PPI use, and quality of life. Results from this meta-analysis, including data from 233 patients, demonstrated that TIF subjects at 3 years had improved esophageal pH, a decreaseu in PPI use, and improved quality of life. Other recent publications are also showing favorable durability with long-term outcomes at 5 years[18,21] and even preliminary data at 10 years.[27]

IS IT SAFE?

Two recent meta-analyses reported that the SAE rate is approximately 2% to 2.5%.[28,29] Huang and colleagues[29] reviewed 16 studies (4 randomized controlled trials [RCTs] and 12 prospective observational trials) reporting 19 SAEs in a total of 781 patients who underwent TIF (2.4%). Incorporating multiple versions of how the procedure has been done over the years (endoluminal fundoplication, TIF 1.0, and TIF 2.0), SAEs included 7 perforations, 5 cases of post-TIF bleeding, 4 cases of pneumothorax, 1 requiring intravenous antibiotics, and 1 involving severe epigastric pain. One death was reported 20 months after the TIF procedure, which was categorized as "probably not related" to the procedure. If, however, one were to exclusively examine the 4 RCTs that prospectively followed adverse events, there was only 1 SAE reported among 188 patients (0.5%), which was a pneumoperitoneum managed with needle decompression. Post-TIF dysphagia can occur transiently in 10% to 18% of patients,[25,30,31] bloating has been reported to occur in 18%,[25,31] and both seem to be self-limited. The overall safety of the procedure has been well established. Since

2008, there have been over 25,000 TIF 2.0 procedures performed, and the reported SAE rate is approximately 0.36% with no mortalities. Although uncommon, the reported SAE's include: esophageal perforation, pleural effusion, mucosal laceration or tear, bleeding, abscess, esophageal laceration, esophageal leak, stomach leak, pneumothorax, pneumoperitoneum, and mediastinitis. Details of these SAEs can be found in the Manufacturer and User Facility Device Experience (MAUDE) FDA database. In our experience, the following steps should be considered in maximizing safety: (1) make sure the procedure is indicated; (2) perform under general anesthesia along with a paralyzing agent; (3) antibiotic prophylaxis (eg, cefazolin 2 g); (4) consider predilation with a savory dilator (54 or 57 Fr) over a guidewire to expand the hypopharynx and the upper esophageal sphincter (not for distal esophagus); and (5) when inserting the device always maintain endoscopic visualization, consider jaw thrust and deflation of endotracheal cuff balloon, gentle left-right rocking motion of the device with forward movement, and stop pushing if force is too great or esophageal deviation is noted at the neck. Once the device is in the stomach, (6) make sure the stomach is well insufflated (using a CO_2 automatic insufflator) before withdrawing the scope into the device and re-advancing through the side port; (7) attempt to screw the helical retractor close to the Z-line (more secure anchor and less mucosal injury); (8) avoid placing fasteners sequentially on top of each other (potential for fistula or leak); (9) when "setting" the device, be mindful of the distance of the GE junction (ex. 40 cm) and visually inspect and avoid the tip of the tissue mold pressing up against the diaphragm; (10) make sure the stomach is well insufflated again before bringing the scope back into the device; and (11) when retracting the device from the esophagus, make sure the helical retractor is visible within the transparent channel, withdraw with a gentle left/right rocking motion, and capitalize on the fact that the scope is positioned in the transparent distal tip of the device—using this as a "window" to inspect the fasteners and any potential tears or breaks in the esophageal mucosa during withdrawal. Always perform a complete endoscopy after the procedure, washing any blood which may obscure a mucosal defect. Mucosal tears can be readily closed with endoscopic clips. Any bleeding encountered is most easily managed by closing the tissue mold over the area for a few minutes of tamponade pressure. Perforations may require endoscopic suturing, stenting, or rescue surgery. Once again, we would reiterate that TIF 2.0 is a very safe procedure—but care and caution should always be exercised to minimize complications.

CONCOMITANT LAPAROSCOPIC HERNIA REPAIR AND TRANSORAL INCISIONLESS FUNDOPLICATION—DOES IT MAKE SENSE?

There continues to be an increased interest in performing TIF along with concomitant laparoscopic hernia repair (cTIF). For surgeons performing both LARS and TIF, the rationale for cTIF includes: (1) a trend moving away from Nissen fundoplication due to higher incidence of postoperative gas/bloat and dysphagia, coupled with established data that TIF produces much less gas/bloat and dysphagia,[32] and emerging data suggesting that cTIF also produces less gas/bloat than traditional LARS;[15,16,33] (2) the nonstandardization of the partial fundoplication (Dor or Toupet); and (3) the concern over future effects of stronger MRI machines on the magnetic sphincter augmentation device.[34]

The LOTUS trial brought to light, in a 5-year randomized, open, parallel-group trial in Europe, that although heartburn and regurgitation were better controlled in the LARS group compared with the esomeprazole group, the patients who underwent surgery had significantly more long-term dysphagia, bloating, and flatulence.[35] The prevalence and severity of symptoms at 5 years in the esomeprazole (266 patients) and LARS groups (248 patients), respectively, were 16% and 8% for heartburn (P = .14), 13% and 2% for acid regurgitation (P<.001), 5% and 11% for dysphagia (P<.001), 28% and 40% for bloating (P<.001), and 40% and 57% for flatulence (P<.001). Experience and data such as these continue to prompt further investigation into procedural strategies that minimize postprocedure side effects while maximizing the therapeutic benefits of LARS.

From a surgical technical point of view, performing an anatomic repair of the hiatal defect alone avoids the more extensive LARS dissection, which may require the creation of a larger retroesophageal window, and the taking down of the short gastric vessels for complete fundic mobilization, which may increase the risk of bleeding and injury to the spleen, and necessitate reposition the bulk of the fundus in the retroesophageal space.

In addition, as mentioned earlier in discussing patient selection, most patients after careful inspection of the GE junction are found to have Hill 3 or above and would benefit from a laparoscopic hernia repair. At this point, if the patient is being evaluated by a gastroenterologist, there seems to be a greater comfort level for the patient who has already established a rapport with this physician, to then schedule a combined procedure with the same gastroenterologist along with the foregut surgeon. Although this is an interesting trend, we currently lack the RCTs needed to establish cTIF efficacy and side effects compared with the standard Nissen or partial fundoplication. However, existing nonrandomized data look promising.

Although the EsophyX device was FDA approved in 2007, the FDA further approved its use in 2017 in patients with hiatal hernias larger than 2 cm in conjunction with laparoscopic hernia repair. In 2011, Ihde and colleagues[15] published a retrospective community-based study evaluating the safety and symptomatic outcomes of a series of 42 patients who had either undergone TIF (24 patients) or cTIF (18 patients) based on the presence of a hiatal hernia 3 cm or larger. There were no long-term postoperative complications. GERD-HRQL scores indicated heartburn elimination in 63% of patients. The need for daily PPI therapy was eliminated in 76% of patients. Atypical symptom relief measured by the median reflux symptom index score reduction was significant (5 [0–47] versus 22 [2–42] on PPIs, P<.001).

In a recent 2-site community study, cTIF was performed in 99 patients with GERD and hiatal hernias between 2 and 5 cm.[33] These patients first underwent a hiatal hernia repair followed immediately by the TIF procedure during the same session. GERD-HRQL, RSI (Reflux Symptom Index), and GERSS (Gastroesophageal Reflux Symptom Score) questionnaires were administered before the procedure and mailed at 6 and 12 months. All patients were symptomatic on PPI medications before cTIF. At 12-month follow-up, median GERD-HRQL scores improved by 17 points, indicating that subjects had no bothersome symptoms. The median GERSS scores decreased from 25.0 at baseline to 1.0, and 90% of subjects reported having effective symptom control (score <18) at 12 months. Seventy-seven percent of subjects reported effective control of laryngopharyngeal reflux symptoms at 12 months with an RSI score of 13 or less. At 12 months, 74% of subjects reported that they were not using PPIs. All measures were statistically improved at P<.05. There were no adverse effects reported. They concluded that cTIF provides significant symptom control for heartburn and regurgitation with no long-term dysphagia or gas bloat normally associated with traditional LARS. Most patients reported durable symptom control and satisfaction with health condition at 12 months.

Although these 2 studies lacked objective esophageal acid exposure data, a more recent study had pre- and post-pH analyses on a subset of patients. In this study by

Idhe and colleagues,[16] 55 patients had cTIF, with 29 patients (53%) having matched preoperative and postoperative validated surveys and pH evaluations. The results showed no serious complications over a mean follow-up of 296 days. The mean GRD HRQL score improved from 33.7 (SD, 22.0) to 9.07 (SD, 13.95) ($P<.001$). The mean RSI score improved from 20.32 (SD, 13) to 8.07 (SD, 9.77) ($P<.001$). The mean pH score improved from 35.3 (SD, 2.27) to 10.9 (SD, 11.5) ($P<.001$). Twenty-two of the 29 patients were judged to have an intact hiatal repair with TIF (76%). Of the 22 patients with an intact hiatal repair and intact fundoplication, 21 (95%) had normalized pH exposure.

Although the emerging data are certainly noteworthy, what remains critically important is more definitive data from randomized control trials with objective outcomes comparing (1) hernia repair plus Nissen fundoplication versus hernia repair plus TIF and (2) hernia repair plus partial fundoplication versus hernia repair plus TIF. These RCTs are currently underway, and hopefully the optimal balance between therapeutic benefits and postprocedural side effects can be carefully weighted.

Not only is TIF now being done concomitantly with laparoscopic hernia repair, but it is also being used as salvage in patients with previous failed LARS. If the failure is with hernia recurrence, we have been performing cTIF for revision. If, however, the failure is with the fundoplication, TIF alone can be an excellent modality to revise the fundoplication without the need for surgery.

WHAT'S NEXT?

With TIF now firmly established as an effective endoscopic antireflux procedure for select patients with GERD, there are many clinical "spaces" where TIF is being explored.

For example, we are now exploring the role of TIF in patients with Barrett's esophagus—including nondysplastic Barrett's—as well as in those patients with a previous history of Barrett's dysplasia who have now reached complete remission of intestinal metaplasia by endoscopic resection and/or ablation, but who are destined to lifelong use of PPIs.

In addition, TIF after per-oral endoscopic myotomy (POEM) is a very exciting area of exploration, because the benefits of POEM over laparoscopic Heller myotomy (LHM) with partial fundoplication for patients with achalasia may be outweighed by the incidence of post-POEM GERD. Recent meta-analyses show that POEM may have better results than LHM[36–39] for improvement of dysphagia, but the issue of post-POEM GERD being higher than post-LHM still needs to be addressed.[40] We need to keep in mind that LHM alone has an incidence of postoperative GERD of approximately 50%, whereas LHM in combination with a partial fundoplication reduces postoperative GERD to approximately 10%.[41] Therefore, most surgeons will automatically perform both operations together. If a substantial number of patients require antireflux surgery after POEM, then it could tip the balance back toward LHM plus partial fundoplication as the preferred first-line option. Fortunately, TIF may represent the endoscopic solution to post-POEM GERD.[42] In our experience of over 60 consecutive POEM procedures, only 3 patients were refractory to PPI medications and the TIF procedure was able to control GERD symptoms and esophagitis in all 3 patients.[43] Further studies examining both efficacy and durability of TIF after POEM are underway. The other consideration between POEM versus LHM plus fundoplication is—whereas the durability of the myotomy (with both POEM and LHM) should be very long, perhaps several decades—the durability of the partial fundoplication may be more limited, probably less than 10 years. At the point of fundoplication loosening, these patients would require either chronic PPI use, a revisional fundoplication, or

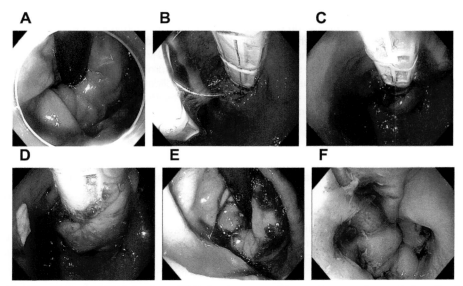

Fig. 17. (A) Pre-TIF Hill 2 Anatomy (B) Retractor secured to greater curve to create length of 3-4cm (C) Approaching lesser curve to create length of 1 to 1.5cm (D) Rotation into anterior corner (E) Completed 4 cm length flap valve (F) Well dispersed fasteners with highest along greater curve (left) and lower along lesser curve (right).

the TIF procedure. Ideally, a POEM with possible TIF in those patients refractory to PPIs will prove effective, as a repeat TIF is much easier to perform than the revision of a fundoplication. There may even be a subset of patients with achalasia who may benefit from concomitant POEM plus TIF in the same procedure. This strategy is being explored in type 1 achalasia patients with dilated and tortuous sigmoid esophagi who may benefit from a preemptive antireflux procedure (much like the LHM plus partial fundoplication strategy), which may also "straighten" the esophagus by retracting more of the esophagus below the diaphragm in creation of the neo valve.

TIF can be considered in obese patients before laparoscopic sleeve gastrectomy (SG), given the higher rate of GERD with SG compared with Roux-En-Y gastric bypass (RYGB).[44–47] Because TIF does not incorporate much of the gastric fundus into the fundoplication, an SG is still feasible after a TIF procedure. This strategy may decrease the number of patients going to RYGB due to preoperative GERD. TIF post-SG is possible, although it requires a sufficient gastric luminal diameter for the device to close (**Fig. 17**).

Finally, there is now a recognized association between lung transplant outcomes and GERD, with data supporting an association between GERD and allograft injury, encouraging a strategy of early diagnosis and aggressive reflux management in lung transplant recipients to improve transplant outcomes.[48,49] There are centers that are currently exploring the role of TIF in the management of these patients.

SUMMARY

GERD is a spectrum disorder, and treatment should be individualized to the anatomic and physiologic alterations of each patient. TIF, as an endoscopic procedure, reduces EGJ distensibility, decreases tLESRs, and creates a 3-cm HPZ at the distal esophagus in the configuration of a flap valve. The gas/bloat side effect is minimized with TIF as it produces a partial fundoplication with a controlled flap valve luminal diameter that allows for venting of the stomach. With proper patient selection, TIF has been shown to be a safe and effective treatment for patients with GERD with hernia less than 2 cm and Hill grade less than 3. The strategy of laparoscopic hernia repair with concomitant TIF is of increasing interest, as are other emerging applications for TIF, such as patients with GERD or Barrett's esophagus, in those after POEM, in those before SG, and even in recipients after lung transplant.

CONFLICT-OF-INTEREST

Dr K.J. Chang has served as consultant for Apollo Endosurgery, Cook, Erbe, Endo-Gastric Solutions, Mauna Kea, Mederi, Medtronics, Olympus, Ovesco, and Pentax.

REFERENCES

1. Richter JE, Rubenstein JH. Presentation and epidemiology of gastroesophageal reflux disease. Gastroenterology 2018;154:267–76.
2. Lord RV, DeMeester SR, Peters JH, et al. Hiatal hernia, lower esophageal sphincter incompetence, and effectiveness of Nissen fundoplication in the spectrum of gastroesophageal reflux disease. J Gastrointest Surg 2009;13:602–10.
3. Tack J, Pandolfino JE. Pathophysiology of gastroesophageal reflux disease. Gastroenterology 2018;154:277–88.
4. Schlottmann F, Andolfi C, Herbella FA, et al. GERD: presence and size of hiatal hernia influence clinical presentation, esophageal function, reflux profile, and degree of mucosal injury. Am Surg 2018;84:978–82.
5. Jobe BA, O'Rourke RW, McMahon BP, et al. Transoral endoscopic fundoplication in the treatment of gastroesophageal reflux disease: the anatomic and physiologic basis for reconstruction of the esophagogastric junction using a novel device. Ann Surg 2008;248:69–76.
6. Rinsma NF, Smeets FG, Bruls DW, et al. Effect of transoral incisionless fundoplication on reflux mechanisms. Surg Endosc 2014;28:941–9.
7. Mittal RK, Zifan A, Kumar D, et al. Functional morphology of the lower esophageal sphincter and crural diaphragm determined by three-dimensional high-resolution esophago-gastric junction pressure profile and CT imaging. Am J Physiol Gastrointest Liver Physiol 2017;313:G212–9.
8. Yassi R, Cheng LK, Rajagopal V, et al. Modeling of the mechanical function of the human gastroesophageal junction using an anatomically realistic three-dimensional model. J Biomech 2009;42:1604–9.
9. Ashfaq A, Rhee HK, Harold KL. Revision of failed transoral incisionless fundoplication by subsequent laparoscopic Nissen fundoplication. World J Gastroenterol 2014;20:17115–9.
10. Bell RC, Cadiere GB. Transoral rotational esophagogastric fundoplication: technical, anatomical, and safety considerations. Surg Endosc 2011;25:2387–99.
11. Barnes WE, Hoddinott KM, Mundy S, et al. Transoral incisionless fundoplication offers high patient satisfaction and relief of therapy-resistant typical and atypical symptoms of GERD in community practice. Surg Innov 2011;18:119–29.
12. Bell RC, Fox MA, Barnes WE, et al. Univariate and multivariate analyses of preoperative factors influencing symptomatic outcomes of transoral fundoplication. Surg Endosc 2014;28:2949–58.

13. Bell RC, Freeman KD. Clinical and pH-metric outcomes of transoral esophago-gastric fundoplication for the treatment of gastroesophageal reflux disease. Surg Endosc 2011;25:1975–84.

14. Chimukangara M, Jalilvand AD, Melvin WS, et al. Long-term reported outcomes of transoral incisionless fundoplication: an 8-year cohort study. Surg Endosc 2019;33:1304–9.

15. Ihde GM, Besancon K, Deljkich E. Short-term safety and symptomatic outcomes of transoral incisionless fundoplication with or without hiatal hernia repair in patients with chronic gastroesophageal reflux disease. Am J Surg 2011;202: 740–6 [discussion: 746–7].

16. Ihde GM 2nd, Pena C, Scitern C, et al. pH scores in hiatal repair with transoral incisionless fundoplication. JSLS 2019;23 [pii:e2018.00087].

17. Narsule CK, Burch MA, Ebright MI, et al. Endoscopic fundoplication for the treatment of gastroesophageal reflux disease: initial experience. J Thorac Cardiovasc Surg 2012;143:228–34.

18. Stefanidis G, Viazis N, Kotsikoros N, et al. Long-term benefit of transoral incisionless fundoplication using the esophyx device for the management of gastroesophageal reflux disease responsive to medical therapy. Dis Esophagus 2017;30:1–8.

19. Testoni PA, Corsetti M, Di Pietro S, et al. Effect of transoral incisionless fundoplication on symptoms, PPI use, and ph-impedance refluxes of GERD patients. World J Surg 2010;34:750–7.

20. Testoni PA, Testoni S, Mazzoleni G, et al. Long-term efficacy of transoral incisionless fundoplication with Esophyx (Tif 2.0) and factors affecting outcomes in GERD patients followed for up to 6 years: a prospective single-center study. Surg Endosc 2015;29:2770–80.

21. Trad KS, Barnes WE, Prevou ER, et al. The TEMPO trial at 5 years: transoral fundoplication (TIF 2.0) is safe, durable, and cost-effective. Surg Innov 2018;25: 149–57.

22. Wilson EB, Barnes WE, Mavrelis PG, et al. The effects of transoral incisionless fundoplication on chronic GERD patients: 12-month prospective multicenter experience. Surg Laparosc Endosc Percutan Tech 2014;24:36–46.

23. Trad KS, Barnes WE, Simoni G, et al. Transoral incisionless fundoplication effective in eliminating GERD symptoms in partial responders to proton pump inhibitor therapy at 6 months: the TEMPO randomized clinical trial. Surg Innov 2015;22: 26–40.

24. Hunter JG, Kahrilas PJ, Bell RC, et al. Efficacy of transoral fundoplication vs omeprazole for treatment of regurgitation in a randomized controlled trial. Gastroenterology 2015;148:324–33.e5.

25. Hakansson B, Montgomery M, Cadiere GB, et al. Randomised clinical trial: transoral incisionless fundoplication vs. sham intervention to control chronic GERD. Aliment Pharmacol Ther 2015;42:1261–70.

26. Gerson L, Stouch B, Lobontiu A. Transoral incisionless fundoplication (TIF 2.0): a meta-analysis of three randomized, controlled clinical trials. Chirurgia (Bucur) 2018;113:173–84.

27. Testoni PA, Distefano G, Mazzoleni G, et al. Transoral incisionless fundoplication with Esophyx (TIF 2.0) for gastro-esophageal reflux disease: three to ten year outcomes in a prospective observational single-center study. Gastrointest Endosc 2018;87:AB 262–263.

28. McCarty TR, Itidiare M, Njei B, et al. Efficacy of transoral incisionless fundoplication for refractory gastroesophageal reflux disease: a systematic review and meta-analysis. Endoscopy 2018;50:708–25.

29. Huang X, Chen S, Zhao H, et al. Efficacy of transoral incisionless fundoplication (TIF) for the treatment of GERD: a systematic review with meta-analysis. Surg Endosc 2017;31:1032–44.

30. Frazzoni M, Conigliaro R, Manta R, et al. Reflux parameters as modified by EsophyX or laparoscopic fundoplication in refractory GERD. Aliment Pharmacol Ther 2011;34:67–75.

31. Witteman BP, Conchillo JM, Rinsma NF, et al. Randomized controlled trial of transoral incisionless fundoplication vs. proton pump inhibitors for treatment of gastroesophageal reflux disease. Am J Gastroenterol 2015;110:531–42.

32. Bazerbachi F, Krishnan K, Abu Dayyeh BK. Endoscopic GERD therapy: a primer for the transoral incisionless fundoplication procedure. Gastrointest Endosc 2019;90(3):370–83.

33. Janu P, Shughoury AB, Venkat K, et al. Laparoscopic hiatal hernia repair followed by transoral incisionless fundoplication with EsophyX device (HH + TIF): efficacy and safety in two community hospitals. Surg Innov 2019;26(6):675–86.

34. Smith CD, Ganz RA, Lipham JC, et al. Lower esophageal sphincter augmentation for gastroesophageal reflux disease: the safety of a modern implant. J Laparoendosc Adv Surg Tech A 2017;27:586–91.

35. Galmiche JP, Hatlebakk J, Attwood S, et al. Laparoscopic antireflux surgery vs esomeprazole treatment for chronic GERD: the LOTUS randomized clinical trial. JAMA 2011;305:1969–77.

36. Schlottmann F, Luckett DJ, Fine J, et al. Laparoscopic heller myotomy versus peroral endoscopic myotomy (POEM) for achalasia: a systematic review and meta-analysis. Ann Surg 2018;267:451–60.

37. Awaiz A, Yunus RM, Khan S, et al. Systematic review and meta-analysis of perioperative outcomes of Peroral Endoscopic Myotomy (POEM) and Laparoscopic Heller Myotomy (LHM) for achalasia. Surg Laparosc Endosc Percutan Tech 2017; 27:123–31.

38. Zhang Y, Wang H, Chen X, et al. Per-oral endoscopic myotomy versus laparoscopic Heller myotomy for achalasia: a meta-analysis of nonrandomized comparative studies. Medicine (Baltimore) 2016;95:e2736.

39. Marano L, Pallabazzer G, Solito B, et al. Surgery or peroral esophageal myotomy for achalasia: a systematic review and meta-analysis. Medicine (Baltimore) 2016; 95:e3001.

40. Repici A, Fuccio L, Maselli R, et al. GERD after per-oral endoscopic myotomy as compared with Heller's myotomy with fundoplication: a systematic review with meta-analysis. Gastrointest Endosc 2018;87:934–943 e18.

41. Richards WO, Torquati A, Holzman MD, et al. Heller myotomy versus Heller myotomy with Dor fundoplication for achalasia: a prospective randomized double-blind clinical trial. Ann Surg 2004;240:405–12 [discussion: 412–5].

42. Tyberg A, Choi A, Gaidhane M, et al. Transoral incisional fundoplication for reflux after peroral endoscopic myotomy: a crucial addition to our arsenal. Endosc Int Open 2018;6:E549–52.

43. Chang KJ. Endoscopic foregut surgery and interventions: the future is now. The state-of-the-art and my personal journey. World J Gastroenterol 2019;25:1–41.

44. Bou Daher H, Sharara AI. Gastroesophageal reflux disease, obesity and laparoscopic sleeve gastrectomy: the burning questions. World J Gastroenterol 2019; 25:4805–13.

45. Gu L, Chen B, Du N, et al. Relationship between bariatric surgery and gastro-esophageal reflux disease: a systematic review and meta-analysis. Obes Surg 2019;29:4105–13.
46. Popescu AL, Ionita-Radu F, Jinga M, et al. Laparoscopic sleeve gastrectomy and gastroesophageal reflux. Rom J Intern Med 2018;56:227–32.
47. Sharples AJ, Mahawar K. Systematic review and meta-analysis of randomised controlled trials comparing long-term outcomes of Roux-En-Y gastric bypass and sleeve gastrectomy. Obes Surg 2019. https://doi.org/10.1007/s11695-019-04235-2.
48. Hathorn KE, Chan WW, Lo WK. Role of gastroesophageal reflux disease in lung transplantation. World J Transplant 2017;7:103–16.
49. Wood RK. Esophageal dysmotility, gastro-esophageal reflux disease, and lung transplantation: what is the evidence? Curr Gastroenterol Rep 2015;17:48.

Innovations in Endoscopic Therapy for Gastroesophageal Reflux Disease

Kara L. Raphael, MD[a], Patrick Walsh, MD[b], Petros C. Benias, MD[a],*

KEYWORDS

- GERD • Endoscopic suturing • Resection • Plication • Lower esophageal sphincter
- Hiatal hernia • Antireflux therapy

KEY POINTS

- Endoscopic antireflux therapy can be considered as a highly effective minimally invasive therapeutic option for patients with GERD without a hiatal hernia.
- Strengthening the distal lower esophageal high-pressure zone is the anatomic and functional goal of endoscopic antireflux therapy.
- Endoscopic suturing techniques that allow for durable full-thickness plications are the most promising endoscopic option to date.
- Full-thickness suturing techniques use simple methods and widely available and low-cost platforms, and can be used on an expanded population of patients with GERD, making this option highly accessible.

 Video content accompanies this article at http://www.giendo.theclinics.com.

IMPACT OF GASTROESOPHAGEAL REFLUX DISEASE

Gastroesophageal reflux disease (GERD) is a widely prevalent condition that can be a detriment to the quality of life of many patients and result in a significant use of health care costs. There have been great strides in our understanding of the pathophysiology of this condition that have driven an evolution of treatments. Today, we continue to rely on proven medical and surgical therapies while we look for newer minimally invasive approaches, such as endoscopic antireflux therapies to bridge the gap.

The prevalence of GERD in the Westernized societies is high and rising, previously estimated to affect up to 20% of the population in the United States,[1,2] but now suspected to be as high as 30%.[3] This prevalence is in line with that of Europe,

Funding Source: None.
[a] Division of Gastroenterology, North Shore-Long Island Jewish Medical Center, Zucker School of Medicine at Hofstra/Northwell, Northwell Health System, Manhasset, NY 11030, USA;
[b] Division of Gastroenterology, St Vincent's Northside Medical Centre, 627 Rode Road, Brisbane, Australia
* Corresponding author.
E-mail address: pbenias@northwell.edu

Gastrointest Endoscopy Clin N Am 30 (2020) 291–307
https://doi.org/10.1016/j.giec.2019.12.009
1052-5157/20/© 2020 Elsevier Inc. All rights reserved.

Australia, and the Middle East, and much higher than in Eastern Asian countries, where GERD only affects up to 5% of the population.[3] GERD does not have a predilection for age or sex,[4] but may have positive associations with smoking,[5] abdominal obesity,[6] *Helicobacter pylori* infections,[7] and the presence of a hiatal hernia.[8] The health care burden associated with this disease is immense; it is estimated that up to $10 billion/year is directly spent in the United States alone, on both diagnostic testing as well as management with prescription medications.[9] Indirect costs as a result of GERD-related absenteeism and work loss are also high, with some studies estimating that cost to employers can range from $500 to $3000 per year for a single employee with GERD.[10] It is imperative to investigate alternative treatments that are minimally invasive, cost-effective, and durable, but to do so we have to have a clear understanding of the GERD patient's underlying anatomy and physiology.

EVALUATION OF THE GASTROESOPHAGEAL JUNCTION

A thorough examination of the gastroesophageal junction (GEJ) is required in the assessment of the patient with GERD. An endoscopic evaluation for a hiatus hernia (HH) is critical, as it is one the main anatomic deficiencies in GERD, and also directs potential intervention. In its simplest form, the hernia is small, nonsliding, and essentially reflects a slightly nonapposing hiatus. These are the HHs that are ideal for endoscopic intervention. In more complex hernias, there is a near complete loss of the phrenoesophageal ligamentous attachments, and a large crural defect results in a significant amount of herniation of the stomach, which poses a significant challenge for endoscopic therapy. However, the ability to classify the HH as large or small can sometimes be difficult to assess because of its sliding nature. In fact, there has been tremendous inconsistency in how we define and report hernias endoscopically, with a bias to under-report small hernias. There have been several studies reporting similar rates of HHs found by endoscopy in Western populations; in Sweden 14.5%,[11] in Norway 16.6%,[12] and in the United States, 22%.[13] In our experience, the true prevalence of an HH is much higher.

An HH should be considered endoscopically significant when the GEJ is positioned at least 2 cm longitudinally above the diaphragmatic orifice. It is also equally as crucial to measure the transverse diaphragmatic defect. To better evaluate the transverse dimension of the hiatal hernia, Hill and colleagues[14] developed a grading scale for the integrity of the GEJ when viewed from a retroflexed position. A widening of the insertion angle of the musculomucosal ridge was associated with a looser flap valve and a higher Hill grade. A higher grade was directly associated with increased reflux symptoms and severity of GERD. One can also simply use the known outer diameter of the endoscope in a retroflexed view to gauge the approximate transverse hiatal diameter in addition to using the Hill grade. One must, therefore, take note of the axial length (>2 cm), transverse diameter (>2 cm), and Hill grade (3 or greater) as a predictor of a large or clinically significant HH. This evaluation is critical, as it is thought that the role of the HH in the pathophysiology of GERD lies primarily in its anatomic disruption of the antireflux barrier.

THE ANTIREFLUX BARRIER

The antireflux barrier is a complex anatomic zone composed of the lower esophageal sphincter (LES), including the gastric sling and clasp fibers, the gastroesophageal flap valve, the crural diaphragm, and the phrenoesophageal membrane. The LES itself is composed of tonically contracted circular smooth muscle at the distal portion of the esophagus, as well as muscular components from the gastric cardia and extrinsic crural diaphragm.[15] The LES offsets backpressure across the GEJ from stomach contents into the esophagus. Subtraction studies using inhibition of the diaphragmatic skeletal muscle versus smooth muscle of the LES shows that the LES has in fact 2 pressure peaks that comprise the lower esophageal high-pressure zone (LEHPZ).[16] The proximal high-pressure zone is made up of the esophageal circular smooth muscle, whereas the distal high-pressure zone seems to be composed of the gastric sling and clasp fibers. High-definition evaluation of this mechanism shows that the gastric sling and clasp fibers crosslink in the left posterior region of the LES, forming what is anatomically referred to as the angle of His. The gastric sling muscle fibers originate from the greater curve of the cardia, and the gastric clasp fibers originate from the lesser curve of the cardia.[16-18] The sling and clasp fibers are stimulated separately but work in concert to form a pressure barrier in the upper stomach.[16] The flap valve is the intraluminal extension of the musculomucosal fold at the angle of His, opposite the lesser curvature of the stomach.[19] As the fundus expands during gastric filling, the fold approximates the lesser curvature, which strengthens the antireflux barrier. Physiologic pressure studies have shown that, in patients with GERD, the distal high-pressure zone composed of these sling-clap fibers seems to be the major deficiency[15] (**Fig. 1**). Relative to the crural diaphragm pressure measurements performed by manometric pull-throughs show that there are 2 peaks, the distal of which is missing in patients with GERD. Whether this is an acquired phenomenon or a key causative observation, it stands as an important target for endoscopic interventions. Other key observations have been that, in patients with GERD, a lower yield or burst pressure is required to distend the flap valve. Such measurements are made by distending the stomach with the intention of compromising the flap valve and directly correlates with the physiology of stomach distention during eating and the postprandial state, which compromises the antireflux apparatus.[20] Therefore, lowering the compliance of the valve would theoretically increase the yield pressures and should increase the threshold at which the valve fails.

The other key component to the antireflux mechanism, the crural diaphragm, is composed of outer craniocaudally directed fibers, and inner obliquely oriented fibers. These work to contract in a "pinchcock"-like action on the LES and act as an extrinsic sphincter at the diaphragmatic hiatus.[21] The diaphragm further interacts with the esophagus by way of ligamentous scaffolding. The phrenoesophageal membrane is the elastic ligamentous organ that affixes the crural diaphragm muscle fibers to the

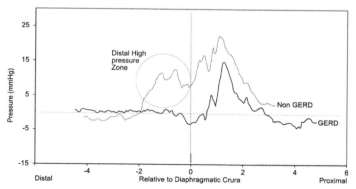

Fig. 1. Representative pressure tracing of GERD versus non-GERD patients relatiuve to crural diaphragm. Patients without GERD have a second distal HPZ, which is absent in patients with GERD. This corresponds to the sling-clasp fibers anatomically.

external portion of the lower esophagus.[22] Thus, it could be surmised that the antireflux barrier is composed of 2 functional components; the internal sphincter action of the LEHPZ, divided into the proximal and distal high-pressure zones, and the extrinsic sphincter action of the crural diaphragm. In fact, this has long been referred to as the "two-sphincter hypothesis."[17]

In the presence of an HH, as the GEJ is displaced above the diaphragmatic hiatus, there is a physical separation of the intrinsic and extrinsic sphincters, a distortion of the flap valve, and a resultant weakening of the LEHPZ. However, GERD is also common in patients without an HH. Despite a lack of a hernia, there are other physiologic deficiencies at play that are crucial as to why these patients develop GERD. It seems as although a deficiency of the distal LEHPZ is the most critical anatomic failure that results in an increased frequency and duration of gastroesophageal reflux events. This deficiency is thought to be caused by a mechanism called transient lower esophageal sphincter relaxations (TLESRs).[23] TLESRs occur when the vagus nerve mediates a stretch-induced neuromuscular inhibition and ultimate transient relaxation of both the LES and the crural diaphragm.[24] They occur independently of swallowing or esophageal peristalsis, last for greater than 10 seconds, and do occur in normal subjects. However, they occur much more frequently in patients with GERD and are thought to be the primary mechanism of gastric reflux in patients without an HH.[25,26]

Restoring the normal anatomy and physiology of the GEJ and antireflux barrier by means of physical hernia reduction has been the goal of surgical therapy for GERD. We can surmise, however, that in patients with GERD and without a significant HH, the distal LEHPZ represents a clear target for intervention. In fact, the patient with little to no evidence of an HH is the ideal candidate for endoscopic antireflux therapy, in which the anatomic goal is to strengthen the LEHPZ and reconstitute the angle of His and the mucosal flap valve.

INTERVENTIONAL THERAPY FOR GASTROESOPHAGEAL REFLUX DISEASE

Historically, surgical Nissen fundoplication has been the mainstay of interventional GERD therapy, reserved for those with partial or nonresponse to medical therapy, as it tightens the LES and repairs the hiatal hernia. Outcomes of multiple randomized controlled trials comparing surgery to medical management were good, with generally high long-term patient satisfaction and decrease of medication use.[27–32] However, postoperative side effects, including dysphagia and bloating, are not uncommon, as well as the need for surgical revision.[33,34] Nissen fundoplications have been found to have a failure rate of up to 30%, primarily due to transdiaphragmatic herniation of the fundoplication, or hernia recurrence. In these cases, reoperation occurs in 5% to 15%, and the second fundoplication has a higher rate of complications.[35–37] To avoid the need for reoperation that is expected to occur in up to one-third of primary surgical patients, less invasive options are increasingly becoming attractive.

One such approach, albeit surgical, is magnetic sphincter augmentation using the LINX system. A ring of magnetic beads is placed laparoscopically at the GEJ, with the goal of increasing LES pressure. This technique has been shown to have less side effects than the Nissen, with a similar improvement in proton pump inhibitor (PPI) use and quality of life.[38–40] However, some studies have shown that the rates of reoperation are similar to the laparoscopic Nissen,[41] and there is a paucity of long-term data at this time.

In terms of endoluminal therapies for GERD, 3 major types have emerged: injection therapy, radiofrequency ablation, and endoscopic suturing. Injection techniques, which focused on endoscopic injection of bulking materials at the GEJ to enhance the antireflux barrier, were initially appealing, but led to a high adverse event rate and were eventually withdrawn from the US market.[42,43] Radiofrequency ablation as with the Stretta device to promote scar tissue formation to tighten the GEJ, as described previously, has had conflicting outcomes data.[44–47] Finally, there have been multiple endoscopic suturing systems and techniques that have been developed over the years with varying degrees of success for GERD therapy. We will now focus this review on previous, current, and future endoscopic suturing and plication techniques.

PREVIOUS ENDOSCOPIC SUTURING THERAPIES

Historically, there have been promising attempts at restoring the mucosal flap valve and augmenting the LES with endoscopic plication. The EndoCinch suturing device was the first such suturing device on the market for the endoscopic treatment of GERD,[48] with the main goal of creating a full-thickness intussusception of the GEJ, resulting in an inverted gastroplication, or in other words, a gastrogastric plication. This plication technique is notable because it improved the Hill grade of the musculomucosal flap valve and reduced the relaxation rate of the LES. Initial studies were quite promising; they showed both an excellent safety profile for EndoCinch as well as efficacy across many measures, including patient symptom scores, reduced PPI use, and improved appearance of the LES.[49–52]

Only a few years after the approval of the EndoCinch device, the NDO Plicator was introduced. This device aimed to create a gastroplication below the GEJ with serosa-to-serosa apposition of the anterior gastric cardia to enhance the flap valve competency. As with the EndoCinch device, follow-up data showed improved esophageal acid exposure in the short-term cohort, and decreased medication use and improved GERD-related symptoms for up to 5 years of follow-up.[53–56] However, despite the apparent success of the device, the Plicator was taken off the market for unclear reasons. Subsequently, an updated and more advanced version of this device, called GERDx, was introduced. Short-term follow-up of patients undergoing gastroplication with the GERDx system showed an acceptable safety profile, improvement in acid exposure, as well as improvement in GERD-related symptoms.[57]

Perhaps the most well-studied suturing device to date has been the EsophyX device for transoral incisionless fundoplication (TIF), which, as described previously, attempts to improve the competency of the antireflux barrier by restoring the angle of His. Five- to 10-year outcomes have been encouraging and comparable with laparoscopic Nissen fundoplication.[58–65] The major limitations, however, continue to be that it is based on a proprietary platform, and it cannot be performed in altered anatomy because of the size of the device, due to the way it is performed in the retroflexed position. In addition, most patients often require an overnight stay. These are the major limitations that suturing for GERD in the *en face* position could potentially eliminate.

OPPORTUNITIES FOR INNOVATION

Despite their fairly successful profiles overall, none of these endoluminal suturing systems or devices are perfect, and some have fallen out of favor. It is helpful to compare the outcomes of the currently available antireflux procedures (**Table 1**). Although the EndoCinch system initially seemed to be a promising minimally invasive therapeutic option for GERD in short-term follow-up, long-term results have been disappointing, with most patients requiring reinitiation of medication and many requiring either retreatment with EndoCinch or referral for laparoscopic fundoplication.[66] The major reason for this is a failure of the plication itself; the infolded mucosa in the plication does not fuse and the sutures often loosen or fall out. Limited ultrasound data suggest

Table 1
Outcomes of the currently available antireflux procedures

Procedure	Procedural Complications	Side Effects	Symptom Reduction (DeMeester or GERD-HRQL Scores)	Elimination or Reduction of PPI Usage	Reflux Events (Reduction in Fraction Time of pH <4)	Reintervention Rate
Nissen	Rare: • Conversion to open surgery • Intraoperative bleeding • Wrap migration • Wrap ischemia • Pneumothorax	Common: • Dysphagia (persistent) • Bloating or gas (persistent) • Inability to belch • Heartburn and regurgitation	Up to 65% of patients at 10 y	Up to 53% of patients at 15 y	Up to 95% of patients at 10 y	Up to 15% of patients
LINX	Rare: • Pleural injury • Intraoperative bleeding • GEJ obstruction • Device erosion	Common: • Postoperative dysphagia (most self-resolve) Rare: • Esophageal spasm	>90% of patients over 2 y	>80% of patients up to 5 y	64%–79% of patients up to 5 y	Up to 3.3% of patients
Stretta	Rare: • Minor postoperative bleeding	Common: • Postoperative chest or abdominal pain	72% of patients at 10 y	64% of patients at 10 y	0%–58% of patients at up to 1 y	Up to 7.3% at 10 y
EndoCinch	Common: • Partial or complete loss of plications at 2 y Rare: • Bleeding from suture site	Rare: • Postoperative dysphagia requiring suture removal	50%–75% of patients at 2 y	45%–69% of patients at 2 y	32%–100% of patients at 2 y	Up to 18% of patients

NDO Plicator	Rare: • Mucosal abrasion	Common: • Postoperative abdominal or chest pain (self-resolved)	0% of patients at 5 y	90% of patients up to 5 y	NR	NR
GERDx	Rare: • Misplaced suture requiring surgical removal	Rare: • Postoperative chest pain	100% of patients at 3 mo	90% of patients at 3 mo	60% of patients at 3 mo	17.5% of patients
TIF	Rare: • Device malfunction	Rare: • Postoperative epigastric pain	>75% of patients at 5 y	Up to 80% of patients at 5 y	40% of patients at 3 y	Up to 7.5% of patients
ARMS	NR	NR	100% of patients at 2 mo	100% of patients at 2 mo	26% of patients at 2 mo	NR
Mucosal augmentation	NR	Rare: • Postoperative nausea & vomiting	100% of patients at 5 mo	20% of patients at 5 mo	NR	NR
MASE	NR	Common: • Postoperative epigastric pain	NR	72% of patients at 4 mo	NR	NR
RAP	NR	Rare: • Stricture requiring dilation	100% of patients at 9 mo	100% of patients at 9 mo	NR	NR

Abbreviations: ARMS, antireflux mucosectomy; NR, not reported; RAP, resection and plication.

that many of these sutures were not in fact full thickness but rather positioned in the submucosa. Loose sutures have been associated with poor efficacy of the plication in up to 50% of patients who underwent EndoCinch procedures.[67,68] The plications made by the GERDx system, as well as the EsophyX device, may also be limited by loose or partial-thickness plications. Further notable limitations include the need for a second endoscopist during the TIF procedure, which may limit its universality, as well as the inability to perform any of these endoscopic procedures in patients with alternate anatomy, as the devices are bulky over the endoscopes and cannot adequately retroflex in small spaces.

Because of these limitations of the current endoscopic antireflux systems, is surgical laparoscopic Nissen fundoplication the better option? When weighing this decision, the risks and complications of surgery need to be carefully considered. Laparoscopic fundoplication carries the risk of long-term morbidity with gas-bloat syndrome, dysphagia, and the need for reintervention, often with another surgery. Clearly, even with the current options in endoscopic and surgical therapies for GERD, there is still a need for a low-cost, widely available, and durable endoscopic option.

CURRENT ADVANCES IN ENDOSCOPIC SUTURING FOR GASTROESOPHAGEAL REFLUX DISEASE

In 2014, Inoue and colleagues[69] published a case series demonstrating that antireflux mucosectomy (ARMS) could be used with success as a treatment for GERD in patients without a hiatal hernia. Initially, this group performed a circumferential endoscopic mucosal resection for treatment of dysplastic Barrett's esophagus, and hypothesized that this technique would also reduce the patient's GERD symptoms by means of the development of a relative stricture from the healed resection at the level of the gastric cardia. In fact, the patient's GERD symptoms were resolved, and the authors next applied this technique to a series of patients with GERD symptoms specifically for this indication. The ARMS technique is to first mark the lesser curvature with an electrocautery knife in a hemicircumferential fashion approximately 2 cm distal from the GEJ, sparing the greater curvature where the mucosal flap valve lies, and 1 cm proximal to the junction into the esophagus. Next, a submucosal injection was performed to lift the mucosa within the marked area. Finally, either an endoscopic mucosa resection or endoscopic submucosal dissection was performed to remove the mucosa. The healing process after mucosectomy involved shrinkage and scarring of this area, which in turn would reduce the gastric cardia opening, sharpen the angle of His, and potentially remodel the flap valve on the opposite site. Indeed, this technique proved effective in their case series of 10 patients; the DeMeester score was significantly reduced, all patients were able to stop PPIs, and the esophageal acid exposure time was also decreased.[69] Several centers subsequently trialed this technique for safety, feasibility, and efficacy, with similar encouraging results, with a good safety profile and over two-thirds of the patients in all studies improving their symptom scores, as well as some decreasing PPI use and improving esophageal acid exposure.[70–72] Although this approach to endoscopic GERD therapy seems promising, because the mucosal resection approach is low cost, it is difficult to deploy on a large scale due to the complexity and technical expertise required to carry out such an extensive resection. Furthermore, larger-scale, comparative, and long-term studies are needed to truly analyze its efficacy and place in the options for endoscopic therapy.

Recently, a novel technique for GERD therapy was developed, born from the need for a simple, cost-effective endoluminal intervention and inspired by the encouraging initial successes of mucosal resection and endoscopic suturing using the Apollo OverStitch device (Apollo Endosurgery, Austin, TX). The theory was that the ease of endoscopic suturing could be enhanced by the durability of scar tissue formation after mucosectomy. This technique is called resection and plication (RAP)[73]. In this procedure, a crescent-shaped (one-third to one-half circumferential) mucosectomy is performed along the greater curvature at the level of the GEJ using a lift and cut technique. As opposed to the lesser curvature location from the ARMS procedure, this mucosectomy was intended to align with the sling fibers, angle of His, and mucosal flap valve. The extent of the mucosectomy was approximately 2 cm in length at the level of the GEJ and just distal to it within the gastric cardia. Next, a full-thickness suture was driven through the exposed muscle fibers of the mucosectomy site in a predetermined suture pattern to tighten the GEJ and create a Hill grade 1 mucosal flap valve (**Fig. 2**). The RAP suturing protocol is meant to recreate a functional valve that would be seen in patients without GERD or a hiatal hernia, allowing for a tightening of the GEJ to reduce reflux events, but importantly does not prevent normal esophageal motility and distensibility. This has been demonstrated by functional cross-sectional area assessments using EndoFLIP measurements (**Fig. 3**). In a pilot study, all patients had a significantly improved GERD symptom score that was sustained over a period of up to 24 months, as well a decreased use of PPI in most (8/10) patients.[73] Again, larger-scale and long-term studies are needed to fully assess the efficacy of this procedure, but these initial results are reassuring.

A procedure similar to RAP, called endoscopic augmentation, has also been evaluated.[74] This technique involves full-thickness endoscopic suturing using the Apollo OverStitch device to narrow the esophageal lumen at the GEJ to reduce reflux exposure. As opposed to RAP, no mucosal resection is used during this technique. An initial study on this technique evaluated 10 patients who had failed or only partially responded to previous therapy (Stretta, TIF, or Nissen fundoplication) who underwent endoscopic reinforcement of the GEJ. A double-channel therapeutic endoscope was used to place individual sutures until a narrowed lumen, traversable with mild-moderate resistance with the double-channel scope, was achieved. A variable number of plications were performed (range 2–8) and was patient specific based on the anatomic appearance. There is, however, a standardized and recommended template for suturing, which in essence creates a trapezoidal-shaped plication along the lesser curvature. All patients had a initial significant reduction in their GERD symptoms scores, although it was reported that this improvement was not sustainable on long-term follow-up.[74]

TECHNIQUE FOR ANTIREFLUX SUTURING

RAP was developed as an amalgam of ARMS and previous suturing techniques to leverage the strength of current full-thickness suturing platforms. It was evident from ARMS that relying on the body's tendency to create scars could result in a durable tightening, thereby augmenting the sling-clasp mechanism. On the other hand, it is not always technically feasible or safe to perform a near 270° endoscopic resection to achieve this on every patient. Finally, allowing the stomach to heal as a result of extensive resection is less predictable than having a templated and predetermined suturing pattern that reshapes the distal valve. Therefore, RAP was developed out of a necessity to use a full-thickness suturing platform.

Resection is a key step for RAP, and appropriate judgment is required as this will create the template for subsequent suturing. In the case of RAP, most resection is

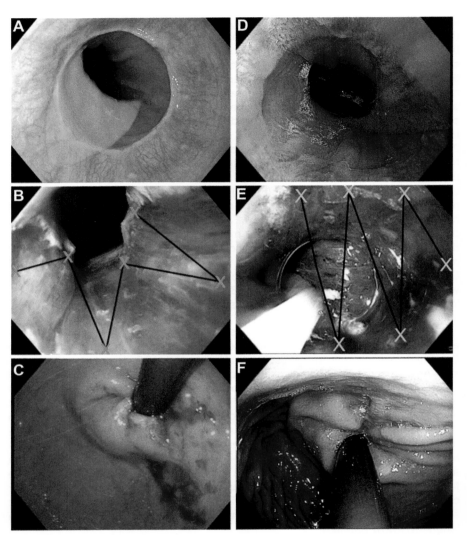

Fig. 2. RAP performed along the greater curvature correlates with the right posterolateral position of the GEJ (A). A predetermined pattern of suturing is used (B) to bring the edges together and achieve a full-thickness plication, which is noted again on retroflexion (C). An aternate approach along the lesser curvature (D) can be used, again with a predetrmined suturing pattern, which differs slightly (E). The retroflexed view (F) differs in its final appearance in that the plication draws the sling fibers down and further accentuates the angle of His.

readily performed with a band ligation kit typically used for mucosal resections or variceal hemostasis. Initial experience with this technique started along the left posterolateral aspect of the GEJ (sling fibers) and has evolved to the right posterolateral aspect (clasp fibers). It is crucial to resect more tissue below the GEJ on the gastric side than above the GEJ lest a stricture is created at the z-line. There have been no head-to-head comparisons between the right versus the left posterolateral aspects; however, there are some differences in

Cross Sectional Area vs Balloon Volume

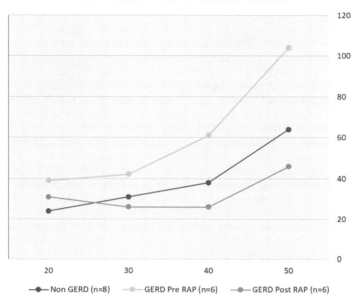

Fig. 3. Cross-sectional area is recorded across various EndoFLIP balloon volumes in healthy volunteers that have normal anatomy and no GERD and in patients with GERD, before RAP and after RAP. EndoFLIP shows that with increasing balloon volumes, normal valves, including those reconstructed by RAP, continue to maintain distensibility, which is not the case with a fixed stricture.

technique and final appearance of the valve. At present, there is not enough data or experience to suggest that one method is superior to the other. On the one hand, greater curvature RAP seems to benefit from a better and more natural scope orientation, easy to perform resection, and more abundant tissue for involution. On the other hand, lesser curvature RAP seems to create a longer flap valve by bolstering the clasp fibers and accentuating the preexisting angle of His (see **Fig. 2**).

If done properly a triangular-shaped mucosal defect is created. Using a band ligator allows the resection to proceed simply and in a regimented manner with little risk of bleeding. Durability is augmented by resection of tissue and application of thermal energy to the submucosal tissue, which is laden with collagen-producing fibroblasts. Again, the aim is to resect up to one-third of the circumference of the GEJ at the level of the z-line, less above and more below. Afterward, the resection base is inspected for bleeding or deeper injury and full-thickness suturing is performed. Suturing usually proceeds from distal to proximal and from right to left. Using the Apollo OverStitch device, a single suture (2 - 0 standard Apollo prolene suture) is directed through the exposed muscle fibers in a full-thickness manner and according to a predetermined pattern.

Herein, the resection also seems to benefit the suturing, in that with the removal of the mucosa, which can be quite thick in this area, it is very clear that the sutures penetrate the muscle consistently. Most cases are performed without the use of a tissue retractor, and only the use of the distal attachment of the suturing system is needed to evert the tissue into the device.

RESECTION AND ABLATION ARE IMPORTANT FOR DURABILITY

Previous attempts at suturing failed due to a lack of a full-thickness suturing system. However, even with such advances in endoscopic technology, it is short sighted to assume that any result will be durable without some impetus for tissue remodeling. Fortinsky and colleagues[75] reported on mucosal ablation and suturing at the esophagogastric junction (MASE) as an evolution of endoscopic augmentation, using argon plasma coagulation to create a more durable result. Similar to the technique of Benias and colleagues,[73] which uses mucosal resection, MASE relies on some level of deeper tissue injury to promote tissue remodeling at the level of the GEJ, which is more durable than the suture alone. Similar to RAP, suturing follows the resection or ablation template. As previously discussed, this area is anatomically under stress and tremendous wear and tear and so most sutures are fated to fail unless they are paired with either ablation, resection, or both. If within the expertise of the endoscopist, it seems that resection may be associated with a better long-term outcome as the reported data on RAP are now at 2 years.[77] Removal of the tissue also allows for deeper transmural suturing, and there does not seem to be a difference in bleeding, an adverse event due to the amount of time the procedure takes to be completed. These techniques have not been compared head-to-head, and the extent to which minor differences between the 2 procedures matters is not clear.

SUTURING IN ALTERNATE ANATOMY

One of the potential benefits of endoscopic suturing for GERD is that it can be performed in an *en face* orientation. Currently, laparoscopic sleeve gastrectomy (LSG) represents a unique and significant challenge as these patients are left with few viable antireflux options. As with most cases of GERD, one needs to take care to exclude other causes of GERD in these patients, such as slight incisural narrowing, which is known to occur in LSG. Apart from this unique situation, however, GERD seems to be prevalent in post-LSG patients, either because of the nature of the population itself or that the LEHPZ is disrupted as the sleeve is created along with mild disruption of the phrenoesophageal ligaments, thereby inherently creating a minor hernia with a weak valve. RAP and MASE have been successfully performed in these patients. For patients with an LSG, a RAP is typically performed along the lesser curvature aspect of the cardia (see **Fig. 2**), since the fundus in these patients has been resected (Video 1).

FUTURE DIRECTIONS

With the resurgence of interest in endoluminal therapy for the treatment of GERD over the last 20 years, many theories, new devices, and protocols have come forward as potentially viable minimally invasive options for the treatment of this widespread disease. Although some techniques have come and gone, others, such as endoscopic suturing, are emerging as promising options. We propose that the use of a widely available, common endoscopic suturing platform, such as Apollo OverStitch, should be the focus of continued investigation and technique development due to its ease of use and initial successes with techniques, such as RAP.

There are multiple areas for further study that are needed to determine the best way to use endoscopic suturing to achieve maximal, sustainable results for GERD therapy. The points of failure in the complex antireflux barrier in the GERD patient should be specifically targeted for correction with endoscopic suturing to best mimic and enhance the normal anatomy. For instance, there should be investigation into the optimal way to recouple the sling and clasp mechanism of the LEHPZ with different suture patterns. The Hill grade and transverse diameter of the GEJ should be reduced as much as possible, without creating an obstruction or disruption of normal esophageal motility. The locations of sutures and surface areas of mucosectomies should be compared to find the best solution for recreating an effective flap valve. Hiatal hernias, which separate the GEJ from the diaphragmatic hiatus and interfere with the two-sphincter barrier mechanism, should be reduced in both transverse and longitudinal diameters. The adequate number and pattern of full-thickness sutures need to be evaluated to determine the most durable but least invasive and time-consuming protocol. Endoscopically, techniques need to be perfected on how to maintain an *en face* working direction, rather than one that requires retroflexion. As endoscopic suturing is highly reliant on the hands of the endoscopist, rather than a standard plication performed by a device, careful training is required so that results are consistent across operators and centers. Finally, well-designed studies that effectively assess both the subjective and objective markers of GERD, as well as appropriate comparisons and long-term follow-up, are a requirement.

Endoscopic suturing is on the precipice of becoming a truly effective minimally invasive therapeutic option for GERD therapy that can rival, and perhaps surpass, the current standards of care given its minimally invasive nature. Continued strategy and innovation into the best method of using this readily available endoscopic tool will push endoscopic suturing into the next chapter of effective endoscopic intervention for GERD.

DISCLOSURE

P.C. Benias is a consultant for Apollo Endosurgery. All other authors indicate no financial disclosures or financial conflicts of interest relevant to this publication.

SUPPLEMENTARY DATA

Supplementary data related to this article can be found online at https://doi.org/10.1016/j.giec.2019.12.009.

REFERENCES

1. Locke GR 3rd, Talley NJ, Fett SL, et al. Prevalence and clinical spectrum of gastroesophageal reflux: a population-based study in Olmsted County, Minnesota. Gastroenterology 1997;112:1448–56.

2. Locke GR 3rd, Talley NJ, Fett SL, et al. Risk factors associated with symptoms of gastroesophageal reflux. Am J Med 1999;106:642–9.

3. El-Serag HB, Sweet S, Winchester CC, et al. Update on the epidemiology of gastro-oesophageal reflux disease: a systematic review. Gut 2014;63:871–80.

4. Becher A, Dent J. Systematic review: ageing and gastro-oesophageal reflux disease symptoms, oesophageal function and reflux oesophagitis. Aliment Pharmacol Ther 2011;33:442–54.

5. Ness-Jensen E, Lagergren J. Tobacco smoking, alcohol consumption and gastro-oesophageal reflux disease. Best Pract Res Clin Gastroenterol 2017;31:501–8.

6. Chang P, Friedenberg F. Obesity and GERD. Gastroenterol Clin North Am 2014;43:161–73.

7. Raghunath A, Hungin AP, Wooff D, et al. Prevalence of *Helicobacter pylori* in patients with gastro-oesophageal reflux disease: systematic review. BMJ 2003; 326:737.

8. Dent J, Becher A, Sung J, et al. Systematic review: patterns of reflux-induced symptoms and esophageal endoscopic findings in large-scale surveys. Clin Gastroenterol Hepatol 2012;10:863–73.e3.

9. Gawron AJ, French DD, Pandolfino JE, et al. Economic evaluations of gastroesophageal reflux disease medical management. Pharmacoeconomics 2014; 32:745–58.

10. Joish VN, Donaldson G, Stockdale W, et al. The economic impact of GERD and PUD: examination of direct and indirect costs using a large integrated employer claims database. Curr Med Res Opin 2005;21:535–44.

11. Cronstedt J, Carling L, Vestergaard P, et al. Oesophageal disease revealed by endoscopy in 1,000 patients referred primarily for gastroscopy. Acta Med Scand 1978;204:413–6.

12. Berstad A, Weberg R, Froyshov Larsen I, et al. Relationship of hiatus hernia to reflux oesophagitis. A prospective study of coincidence, using endoscopy. Scand J Gastroenterol 1986;21:55–8.

13. Wright RA, Hurwitz AL. Relationship of hiatal hernia to endoscopically proved reflux esophagitis. Dig Dis Sci 1979;24:311–3.

14. Hill LD, Kozarek RA, Kraemer SJ, et al. The gastroesophageal flap valve: in vitro and in vivo observations. Gastrointest Endosc 1996;44:541–7.

15. Brasseur JG, Ulerich R, Dai Q, et al. Pharmacological dissection of the human gastro-oesophageal segment into three sphincteric components. J Physiol 2007;580:961–75.

16. Miller L, Vegesna A, Ruggieri M, et al. Normal and abnormal physiology, pharmacology, and anatomy of the gastroesophageal junction high-pressure zone. Ann N Y Acad Sci 2016;1380:48–57.

17. Winans CS. Manometric asymmetry of the lower-esophageal high-pressure zone. Am J Dig Dis 1977;22:348–54.

18. Liebermann-Meffert D, Allgower M, Schmid P, et al. Muscular equivalent of the lower esophageal sphincter. Gastroenterology 1979;76:31–8.

19. Thor KB, Hill LD, Mercer DD, et al. Reappraisal of the flap valve mechanism in the gastroesophageal junction. A study of a new valvuloplasty procedure in cadavers. Acta Chir Scand 1987;153:25–8.

20. Pandolfino JE, Shi G, Curry J, et al. Esophagogastric junction distensibility: a factor contributing to sphincter incompetence. Am J Physiol Gastrointest Liver Physiol 2002;282:G1052–8.

21. Mittal RK, Balaban DH. The esophagogastric junction. N Engl J Med 1997;336: 924–32.

22. Daniels BT. The phrenoesophageal membrane. Am J Surg 1965;110:814–7.

23. Tack J, Pandolfino JE. Pathophysiology of gastroesophageal reflux disease. Gastroenterology 2018;154:277–88.

24. Mittal RK, Holloway RH, Penagini R, et al. Transient lower esophageal sphincter relaxation. Gastroenterology 1995;109:601–10.

25. Miller LS, Vegesna AK, Brasseur JG, et al. The esophagogastric junction. Ann N Y Acad Sci 2011;1232:323–30.

26. Miller L, Vegesna A, Kalra A, et al. New observations on the gastroesophageal antireflux barrier. Gastroenterol Clin North Am 2007;36:601–17, ix.

27. Anvari M, Allen C, Marshall J, et al. A randomized controlled trial of laparoscopic nissen fundoplication versus proton pump inhibitors for treatment of patients with

chronic gastroesophageal reflux disease: one-year follow-up. Surg Innov 2006; 13:238–49.

28. Mahon D, Rhodes M, Decadt B, et al. Randomized clinical trial of laparoscopic Nissen fundoplication compared with proton-pump inhibitors for treatment of chronic gastro-oesophageal reflux. Br J Surg 2005;92:695–9.

29. Lundell L, Miettinen P, Myrvold HE, et al. Long-term management of gastro-oesophageal reflux disease with omeprazole or open antireflux surgery: results of a prospective, randomized clinical trial. The Nordic GORD Study Group. Eur J Gastroenterol Hepatol 2000;12:879–87.

30. Lundell L, Attwood S, Ell C, et al. Comparing laparoscopic antireflux surgery with esomeprazole in the management of patients with chronic gastro-oesophageal reflux disease: a 3-year interim analysis of the LOTUS trial. Gut 2008;57:1207–13.

31. Ciovica R, Gadenstatter M, Klingler A, et al. Quality of life in GERD patients: medical treatment versus antireflux surgery. J Gastrointest Surg 2006;10:934–9.

32. Mehta S, Bennett J, Mahon D, et al. Prospective trial of laparoscopic nissen fundoplication versus proton pump inhibitor therapy for gastroesophageal reflux disease: seven-year follow-up. J Gastrointest Surg 2006;10:1312–6 [discussion: 1316–7].

33. Dallemagne B, Weerts J, Markiewicz S, et al. Clinical results of laparoscopic fundoplication at ten years after surgery. Surg Endosc 2006;20:159–65.

34. Yates RB, Oelschlager BK. Surgical treatment of gastroesophageal reflux disease. Surg Clin North Am 2015;95:527–53.

35. Hunter JG, Smith CD, Branum GD, et al. Laparoscopic fundoplication failures: patterns of failure and response to fundoplication revision. Ann Surg 1999;230: 595–604 [discussion: 604–6].

36. Del Campo SEM, Mansfield SA, Suzo AJ, et al. Laparoscopic redo fundoplication improves disease-specific and global quality of life following failed laparoscopic or open fundoplication. Surg Endosc 2017;31:4649–55.

37. Furnee EJ, Draaisma WA, Broeders IA, et al. Surgical reintervention after failed antireflux surgery: a systematic review of the literature. J Gastrointest Surg 2009;13:1539–49.

38. Aiolfi A, Asti E, Bernardi D, et al. Early results of magnetic sphincter augmentation versus fundoplication for gastroesophageal reflux disease: systematic review and meta-analysis. Int J Surg 2018;52:82–8.

39. Skubleny D, Switzer NJ, Dang J, et al. LINX((R)) magnetic esophageal sphincter augmentation versus Nissen fundoplication for gastroesophageal reflux disease: a systematic review and meta-analysis. Surg Endosc 2017;31:3078–84.

40. Zadeh J, Andreoni A, Treitl D, et al. Spotlight on the Linx Reflux Management System for the treatment of gastroesophageal reflux disease: evidence and research. Med Devices (Auckl) 2018;11:291–300.

41. Guidozzi N, Wiggins T, Ahmed AR, et al. Laparoscopic magnetic sphincter augmentation versus fundoplication for gastroesophageal reflux disease: systematic review and pooled analysis. Dis Esophagus 2019;32(9) [pii:doz031].

42. O'Connor KW, Lehman GA. Endoscopic placement of collagen at the lower esophageal sphincter to inhibit gastroesophageal reflux: a pilot study of 10 medically intractable patients. Gastrointest Endosc 1988;34:106–12.

43. Fockens P, Cohen L, Edmundowicz SA, et al. Prospective randomized controlled trial of an injectable esophageal prosthesis versus a sham procedure for endoscopic treatment of gastroesophageal reflux disease. Surg Endosc 2010;24: 1387–97.

44. Liang WT, Wu JM, Wang F, et al. Stretta radiofrequency for gastroesophageal reflux disease-related respiratory symptoms: a prospective 5-year study. Minerva Chir 2014;69:293–9.

45. Dughera L, Rotondano G, De Cento M, et al. Durability of Stretta radiofrequency treatment for GERD: results of an 8-year follow-up. Gastroenterol Res Pract 2014; 2014:531907.

46. Noar M, Squires P, Noar E, et al. Long-term maintenance effect of radiofrequency energy delivery for refractory GERD: a decade later. Surg Endosc 2014;28: 2323–33.

47. Arts J, Bisschops R, Blondeau K, et al. A double-blind sham-controlled study of the effect of radiofrequency energy on symptoms and distensibility of the gastro-esophageal junction in GERD. Am J Gastroenterol 2012;107:222–30.

48. Swain CP, Mills TN. An endoscopic sewing machine. Gastrointest Endosc 1986; 32:36–8.

49. Schwartz MP, Wellink H, Gooszen HG, et al. Endoscopic gastroplication for the treatment of gastro-oesophageal reflux disease: a randomised, sham-controlled trial. Gut 2007;56:20–8.

50. Liu JJ, Glickman JN, Carr-Locke DL, et al. Gastroesophageal junction smooth muscle remodeling after endoluminal gastroplication. Am J Gastroenterol 2004; 99:1895–901.

51. Chen YK, Raijman I, Ben-Menachem T, et al. Long-term outcomes of endoluminal gastroplication: a U.S. multicenter trial. Gastrointest Endosc 2005;61:659–67.

52. Ozawa S, Kumai K, Higuchi K, et al. Short-term and long-term outcome of endo-luminal gastroplication for the treatment of GERD: the first multicenter trial in Japan. J Gastroenterol 2009;44:675–84.

53. Pleskow D, Rothstein R, Lo S, et al. Endoscopic full-thickness plication for the treatment of GERD: a multicenter trial. Gastrointest Endosc 2004;59:163–71.

54. Pleskow D, Rothstein R, Lo S, et al. Endoscopic full-thickness plication for the treatment of GERD: 12-month follow-up for the North American open-label trial. Gastrointest Endosc 2005;61:643–9.

55. Pleskow D, Rothstein R, Kozarek R, et al. Endoscopic full-thickness plication for the treatment of GERD: long-term multicenter results. Surg Endosc 2007;21: 439–44.

56. Pleskow D, Rothstein R, Kozarek R, et al. Endoscopic full-thickness plication for the treatment of GERD: five-year long-term multicenter results. Surg Endosc 2008;22:326–32.

57. Weitzendorfer M, Spaun GO, Antoniou SA, et al. Clinical feasibility of a new full-thickness endoscopic plication device (GERDx) for patients with GERD: results of a prospective trial. Surg Endosc 2018;32:2541–9.

58. Witteman BP, Strijkers R, de Vries E, et al. Transoral incisionless fundoplication for treatment of gastroesophageal reflux disease in clinical practice. Surg Endosc 2012;26:3307–15.

59. Huang X, Chen S, Zhao H, et al. Efficacy of transoral incisionless fundoplication (TIF) for the treatment of GERD: a systematic review with meta-analysis. Surg Endosc 2017;31:1032–44.

60. Muls V, Eckardt AJ, Marchese M, et al. Three-year results of a multicenter pro-spective study of transoral incisionless fundoplication. Surg Innov 2013;20: 321–30.

61. Testoni PA, Testoni S, Mazzoleni G, et al. Long-term efficacy of transoral incision-less fundoplication with Esophyx (Tif 2.0) and factors affecting outcomes in

GERD patients followed for up to 6 years: a prospective single-center study. Surg Endosc 2015;29:2770–80.

62. Trad KS, Fox MA, Simoni G, et al. Transoral fundoplication offers durable symptom control for chronic GERD: 3-year report from the TEMPO randomized trial with a crossover arm. Surg Endosc 2017;31:2498–508.

63. Trad KS, Barnes WE, Prevou ER, et al. The TEMPO trial at 5 years: transoral fundoplication (TIF 2.0) is safe, durable, and cost-effective. Surg Innov 2018;25: 149–57.

64. Stefanidis G, Viazis N, Kotsikoros N, et al. Long-term benefit of transoral incisionless fundoplication using the EsophyX device for the management of gastroesophageal reflux disease responsive to medical therapy. Dis Esophagus 2017;30:1–8.

65. Testoni PA, Testoni S, Distefano G, et al. Transoral incisionless fundoplication with EsophyX for gastroesophageal reflux disease: clinical efficacy is maintained up to 10 years. Endosc Int Open 2019;7:E647–54.

66. Schwartz MP, Schreinemakers JR, Smout AJ. Four-year follow-up of endoscopic gastroplication for the treatment of gastroesophageal reflux disease. World J Gastrointest Pharmacol Ther 2013;4:120–6.

67. Schiefke I, Zabel-Langhennig A, Neumann S, et al. Long term failure of endoscopic gastroplication (EndoCinch). Gut 2005;54:752–8.

68. Arts J, Lerut T, Rutgeerts P, et al. A one-year follow-up study of endoluminal gastroplication (Endocinch) in GERD patients refractory to proton pump inhibitor therapy. Dig Dis Sci 2005;50:351–6.

69. Inoue H, Ito H, Ikeda H, et al. Anti-reflux mucosectomy for gastroesophageal reflux disease in the absence of hiatus hernia: a pilot study. Ann Gastroenterol 2014;27:346–51.

70. Yoo IK, Ko WJ, Kim HS, et al. Anti-reflux mucosectomy using a cap-assisted endoscopic mucosal resection method for refractory gastroesophageal disease: a prospective feasibility study. Surg Endosc 2019. https://doi.org/10.1007/s00464-019-06859-y.

71. Ota K, Takeuchi T, Harada S, et al. A novel endoscopic submucosal dissection technique for proton pump inhibitor-refractory gastroesophageal reflux disease. Scand J Gastroenterol 2014;49:1409–13.

72. Hedberg HM, Kuchta K, Ujiki MB. First experience with banded anti-reflux mucosectomy (ARMS) for GERD: feasibility, safety, and technique (with video). J Gastrointest Surg 2019;23:1274–8.

73. Benias PC, D'Souza L, Lan G, et al. Initial experience with a novel resection and plication (RAP) method for acid reflux: a pilot study. Endosc Int Open 2018;6: E443–9.

74. Han J, Chin M, Fortinsky KJ, et al. Endoscopic augmentation of gastroesophageal junction using a full-thickness endoscopic suturing device. Endosc Int Open 2018;6:E1120–5.

75. Fortinsky KJ, Shimizu T, Chin MA, et al. Tu1168 Mucosal Ablation And Suturing at the Esophagogastric Junction (MASE): A novel procedure for the management of patients with Gastroesophageal Reflux Disease. Gastrointest Endosc 2018;87(6 Supplement):AB552.

Laparoscopic Hernia Repair and Fundoplication for Gastroesophageal Reflux Disease

Steven R. DeMeester, MD

KEYWORDS

- Fundoplication • Hiatal hernia • Antireflux surgery

KEY POINTS

- The Nissen fundoplication has stood the test of time and has evolved from open laparotomy or thoracotomy to a minimally invasive laparoscopic approach with a short hospital stay, rapid return to normal activities, and minimal perioperative morbidity. It remains the gold standard for the durable relief of gastroesophageal reflux disease (GERD) symptoms and esophagitis.
- The degree of a fundoplication can be tailored, and, in patients with early reflux disease, such as those with heartburn or regurgitation symptoms without esophageal damage, a partial fundoplication offers fewer side effects and may be the preferred approach. Alternatively, the magnetic sphincter augmentation device or an endoscopic antireflux procedure may be ideal in patients with little or no hiatal hernia and early reflux disease.
- All antireflux procedures have a failure rate, and it is important to understand factors that are associated with failure and minimize them to ensure optimal outcomes in patients that present for antireflux surgery. A failed antireflux procedure is troublesome for the patient, can lead to worse reflux disease than the patient had before the procedure, and is a risk factor for progression in patients with Barrett's esophagus.
- The selection of patients for antireflux surgery as well as the choice of the procedure, be it a fundoplication, the magnetic sphincter augmentation device, or an endoscopic approach, requires a thorough understanding of esophageal physiology and the pros and cons of various options. It is best done by focused foregut surgeons that maintain a high volume of procedures and can offer all available options to patients with GERD and guide patients to the best procedure for their disease stage and expectations.

HISTORICAL OVERVIEW

Treatment of gastroesophageal reflux disease (GERD) has changed markedly over the last half century. Before the introduction of H_2 blockers in the 1980s, medical therapy for GERD consisted of antacids and offered poor symptom relief. Even though surgical

Thoracic and Foregut Surgery, General and Minimally Invasive Surgery, The Oregon Clinic, 4805 Northeast Glisan Street, Suite 6N60, Portland, OR 97213, USA
E-mail address: sdemeester@orclinic.com

Gastrointest Endoscopy Clin N Am 30 (2020) 309–324
https://doi.org/10.1016/j.giec.2019.12.007
1052-5157/20/© 2020 Elsevier Inc. All rights reserved.

giendo.theclinics.com

therapy at that time was done via open laparotomy or thoracotomy, highly symptomatic patients with GERD elected to undergo surgery to achieve relief from their severe heartburn and regurgitation symptoms. Early surgical therapies were designed to correct the anatomic defects of a hiatal hernia. Later, a fundoplication was added to increase the efficacy of reflux control. The introduction of H_2 blockers and then proton pump inhibitors (PPIs) provided much more effective medical therapy for GERD symptoms, and although antireflux surgery had progressed to being done in a minimally invasive fashion, the number of patients referred or considered for antireflux surgery was declining by the end of the twentieth century. Now, in the twenty-first century, concern regarding the potential long-term side effects of PPIs, as well as a realization that many patients with GERD are not satisfied with their symptom control on medical therapy, has prompted renewed interest in surgical intervention for GERD. This interest has been further bolstered by new endoscopic and minimally invasive surgical options to restore competency to the lower esophageal sphincter (LES). In addition, decades of research have led to a far better understanding of the pathophysiology of GERD. The challenge of antireflux surgery now is to use the understanding of GERD pathophysiology to provide focused, individualized antireflux interventions that maximize the likelihood of symptom relief while minimizing the potential for side effects or complications.

FUNDOPLICATIONS

The traditional surgical procedure for GERD is a fundoplication, which entails taking the fundus of the stomach and wrapping (or plicating; ergo fundoplication) it to various degrees around the distal esophagus. A complete 360° wrap is known as a Nissen fundoplication. There are numerous forms of partial fundoplication, all of which are characterized by something less than a 360° wrap of the fundus around the esophagus. The most common partial anterior fundoplication is called a Dor, or, when done transthoracically, a Belsey mark IV, whereas the most common partial posterior fundoplication is called a Toupet. Regardless of the type of fundoplication, the mechanism of action depends on several factors: (1) reconstruction of the geometric relationships normally present in the distal esophagus and gastroesophageal junction (GEJ), namely recreation of the angle of His and appropriate positioning of the LES within the crural diaphragm; (2) restoration of LES competency by reestablishing pressure and length; and (3) placement of an adequate length of the LES in the positive pressure environment of the abdomen.[1] To accomplish these objectives during antireflux surgery, any associated hiatal hernia must be repaired, adequate intra-abdominal esophageal length must be established, and the fundoplication must be properly positioned around the distal esophagus over the region of the LES.

The importance of each of these objectives has been confirmed over the 6 decades that antireflux surgery has been performed. Early in the experience with laparoscopic fundoplications, some surgeons did not repair the hiatal hernia and significantly worse outcomes were reported.[1] This experiment has been repeated again with both the introduction of the magnetic sphincter augmentation (LINX) device and the transoral incisionless fundoplication (TIF) procedure. Again, the outcomes in patients with hiatal hernias that were not repaired were inferior to those with no hernia or in whom the hiatal hernia was repaired at the time of device implantation.[2,3] The necessity of an adequate intra-abdominal length of esophagus was established early and led to the development of the Collis gastroplasty in 1957.[4] Recent retrospective studies have suggested a decreased recurrence rate when an adequate intra-abdominal esophageal length is established at the time of antireflux surgery.[5] Lastly, the addition of a fundoplication has been shown to lead to improved outcomes compared with repair of the hiatal hernia alone. The concept of hiatal hernia repair alone was explored by Allison[6,7] in the 1950s, but in 1973 he reported a high frequency of reflux disease in these patients. Others have confirmed these findings in a randomized trial.[8] Consequently, all 3 components (hiatal hernia repair, obtaining an adequate length of intra-abdominal esophagus, and the addition of a fundoplication that is properly positioned around the distal esophagus) are critical for obtaining optimal patient outcomes with an antireflux operation.

Another important principle related to antireflux surgery is that, in contrast with surgical procedures in which an organ is removed, such as appendectomy or cholecystectomy, antireflux surgery is reconstructive surgery designed to correct anatomic and physiologic defects rather than remove the damaged or diseased organ. As such, antireflux surgery is very technique dependent, and variations in the technique between surgeons and centers can alter the outcome of the procedure. For example, although a Nissen is a 360° fundoplication, which part of the fundus and how many sutures are used to make the fundoplication often differ among surgeons. To make matters worse, some surgeons call any fundoplication a Nissen, regardless of whether the fundoplication is a full 360°. Consequently, it is important for anyone caring for a patient after antireflux surgery to understand what type of fundoplication was done as well as the important technical details of the procedure. This requirement is particularly important if the patient is having dysphagia or other postoperative symptoms, or has had a failed fundoplication and revisional surgery is being considered.

TAILORED FUNDOPLICATION

The concept of a tailored fundoplication is that the fundoplication is individualized based on patient factors such as esophageal motility and the severity of GERD. It would seem ideal if only 1 type of fundoplication was used, and that this fundoplication was as standardized as possible to minimize variation between surgeons and centers and produce a reliably excellent outcome. There are surgeons that suggest that a Nissen can and should be used in all patients.[9,10] In the study by Patti and colleagues[10] there were 235 patients that had a tailored approach with either a partial or total fundoplication depending on the results of preoperative manometry, and 122 subsequent patients that all had a total fundoplication regardless of the preoperative manometry findings. There was no difference in the frequency of postoperative dysphagia between groups. Further, reflux control was better in the total fundoplication group. The investigators concluded that a Nissen fundoplication was preferred for all patients with GERD regardless of preoperative esophageal body function on manometry. Importantly, in this study poor motility was defined as esophageal body amplitudes of contraction less than 40 mm Hg and patients with scleroderma were excluded.[10]

Despite these articles, there are several reasons to consider tailoring the fundoplication, or individualizing the degree of the fundoplication to the patient rather than taking a 1-size fits all (ie, Nissen for everybody) approach. First, there clearly is a threshold level of dysmotility at which a Nissen fundoplication provides too much outflow resistance and leads to a high rate of dysphagia. This threshold level has been shown in patients with achalasia who had a Nissen fundoplication with myotomy.[11] The outflow resistance of a Nissen is approximately 20 mm Hg and, therefore, if the esophageal body has amplitudes of contraction in the range of 30 mm Hg or more it is likely that a Nissen fundoplication would be tolerated. However, in patients with ineffective esophageal motility and amplitudes of contraction closer to 20 mm Hg, dysphagia may be a significant problem if a Nissen or 360° fundoplication is constructed.[12] In contrast, partial fundoplications are associated with a lower frequency of dysphagia and are tolerated even in patients with achalasia.[11] The first reason to tailor a fundoplication is therefore to minimize the risk of protracted dysphagia in patients with poor esophageal motility.

The second reason to tailor a fundoplication is based on the preoperative severity of GERD. There is substantial evidence that the objective control of reflux, as determined with postoperative pH testing, is related to the degree of the fundoplication, with the best control by a complete 360° Nissen fundoplication.[10] Further, there is evidence that long-term durability, particularly in patients with preoperative severe reflux disease, is better with a Nissen fundoplication than a partial fundoplication.[13] Consequently, in patients with advanced reflux disease, such as those with Los Angeles grade C or D esophagitis, long-segment Barrett's esophagus, or pulmonary disease from recurrent aspiration events related to reflux, a Nissen fundoplication is preferred to provide the most reliable control of GERD. A Nissen fundoplication reliably abolishes reflux of gastric juice into the esophagus. Commonly, pH testing after a Nissen fundoplication shows none or almost no episodes of reflux over 24 or 48 hours. However, along with maximal control of reflux comes the potential for postfundoplication side effects. Although these side effects can occur with any fundoplication, the frequency and severity may be increased with a Nissen compared with a partial fundoplication. Consequently, in patients with less severe reflux disease, the side effect profile of a Nissen may prove excessive and these patients may be best served with a partial fundoplication.

The last concept about tailoring is that currently antireflux surgery options are not limited to a Nissen or partial fundoplication. Instead, there is magnetic sphincter augmentation with the LINX device, TIF, and other endoscopic interventions under investigation. Consequently, the concept of tailoring should extend to the choice of the type of procedure rather than just the type of fundoplication. The challenge of modern antireflux surgery is to match the best procedure to the individual patient based on multiple preoperative factors, including severity of disease; presence and size of a hiatal hernia; esophageal function; status of the LES; mucosal damage in the esophagus; and patient wishes for the outcome of the procedure in terms of the balance of reflux control, expected longevity of the procedure, and postprocedure side effects.

POSTFUNDOPLICATION SIDE EFFECTS

A fundoplication of any type is designed to restrict the backflow of gastric contents into the esophagus. It does this by increasing the resting pressure of the LES, increasing the residual pressure or the integrated residual pressure during LES relaxation, and increasing the yield pressure of the LES in the setting of gastric distension. These alterations stop reflux of all types: acid, weak acid, alkaline, and bile reflux. Consequently, a fundoplication has some expected side effects, particularly the inability to belch or vomit and increased flatulence. Most patients cannot vomit through an intact wrap, although this is rarely clinically relevant. Importantly, because of this any patient that develops evidence of a bowel obstruction after a fundoplication should promptly be treated with a nasogastric tube to avoid a closed-loop obstruction. Hyperflatulence is a common and noticeable side effect, likely related to more frequent swallowing, which is present in most patients with reflux disease, and to some degree so-called power swallowing early after the fundoplication to overcome the resistance of the new fundoplication.

Dysphagia is a postfundoplication side effect that has received a lot of attention. What is not well appreciated is that dysphagia is a common preoperative symptom and is related to the severity of preoperative reflux disease.[14] Importantly, most preoperative dysphagia resolves after elimination of reflux with a fundoplication.[14] In the first month after a fundoplication, dysphagia is expected related to postoperative swelling. This dysphagia is temporary and typically resolves by 6 to 12 weeks after surgery. During the time when edema is present, patients are instructed to take a graduated diet moving up to soft foods. Thereafter, patients resume a regular diet and can eat things that they often were unable to because of the reflux symptoms those foods produced before their surgery. Patients are counseled to take their time during meals because the fundoplication acts as a "speed bump" in the distal esophagus. The typical American pattern of eating a large quantity of food rapidly does not work well after antireflux surgery, and is not a healthy eating pattern. Instead, a more European eating style (smaller meals eaten slowly) is better and allows most patients to eat comfortably without dysphagia after a fundoplication. Persistent dysphagia beyond 3 to 6 months after a fundoplication is uncommon and warrants evaluation with barium upper gastrointestinal study and upper endoscopy with possible dilatation. A dilatation seldom affects the fundoplication but improves dysphagia related to a stricture in the esophagus or a tight crural closure.

Another potential postfundoplication side effect is gas bloat. Bloat can occur because patients are unable to belch and vent a distended stomach after a fundoplication. This problem can be exacerbated by significantly delayed gastric emptying. However, a fundoplication improves gastric emptying, and this offsets gas bloat symptoms in some patients.[15] The improvement in gastric emptying that accompanies use of the fundus for the construction of the fundoplication is related to the fundus being the part of the stomach involved in the receptive relaxation that allows accommodation of a large meal. Use of a portion of the fundus leads to improved gastric emptying after fundoplication. In extreme cases, some patients benefit from a temporary gastrostomy tube to allow venting of the stomach. Often within a month or two these patients no longer need the tube and it can be removed.

Important concepts about so-called postfundoplication symptoms are that they are common in patients with reflux disease on medical therapy, when present after antireflux surgery they are seldom severe, and the frequency and severity may be reduced in patients with a partial compared with a total fundoplication. A randomized trial between esomeprazole and antireflux surgery showed that dysphagia and flatulence were present in both treatment arms before and after therapy. The frequency was higher after antireflux surgery, but in most patients was considered mild or moderate. In contrast, heartburn and regurgitation symptoms were worse in the medical therapy arm during follow-up.[16] In another randomized trial that compared omeprazole with antireflux surgery the prevalence of posttreatment dysphagia was 5% to 15% in the surgical arm versus 2% to 7% in the medical arm. Flatulence was present in 40% to 70% of patients in the surgery arm compared with 40% in the medical arm, and impaired ability to belch in 15% to 25% after surgery compared with 2% to 10% on medical therapy.[17] There is evidence that the frequency and perhaps severity of postfundoplication side effects are reduced in patients that have a partial compared with a total fundoplication.[18] However, the difference seems to lessen with time. In a prospective, randomized trial from Australia, patients that had a laparoscopic Nissen fundoplication were compared with those that had a partial, anterior 180° fundoplication. At a mean follow-up of 10 years, there were no significant differences in reflux symptoms, dysphagia, abdominal bloating, ability to belch, or overall satisfaction between the 2 groups.[19] Thus, although much is made of postfundoplication symptoms, the data suggest they are seldom severe, occur in a minority of patients, dissipate with time, and are present in many patients on medical therapy for their GERD.

CANDIDATES FOR ANTIREFLUX SURGERY

Anyone with objectively proven GERD is a potential candidate for antireflux surgery, and it may be the preferred option in younger patients, those who are noncompliant or concerned about the long-term side effects of PPI medications, those for whom medications are a financial burden, those who have incomplete symptom relief with medications, and those who favor a single intervention rather than long-term drug treatment. Further, there is increasing support for the application of an antireflux procedure in patients at risk for progressive disease.[20] Risk factors for progressive disease in patients with GERD are still being elucidated but include nocturnal reflux on 24-hour esophageal pH study, a structurally deficient LES, mixed reflux of gastric and duodenal juice, esophagitis at presentation or esophagitis that persists after initial acid-suppression therapy, a family history of GERD, regular alcohol intake, and regular use of PPI medications.[21,22]

Because antireflux surgery abolishes all types of reflux (acid, weak acid, and alkaline), it provides reliable relief of GERD, but only if the symptoms are caused by GERD. However, even the classic GERD symptoms of heartburn and regurgitation are not always caused by increased esophageal acid exposure, and there are numerous cases of antireflux surgery being done in patients with achalasia or other disorders misdiagnosed as GERD based largely on a symptomatic assessment preoperatively. Because the anticipated success rate of laparoscopic fundoplication is directly proportional to the degree of certainty that GERD is the underlying cause of the patient's complaints, GERD should be confirmed with objective studies, and performing an antireflux operation because of symptoms alone should be avoided. Objective methods to confirm GERD include confirming increased esophageal acid exposure on pH testing, an upper endoscopy showing LA grade C or D esophagitis, or a columnar-lined esophagus with intestinal metaplasia on biopsy (Barrett's esophagus).[23] Impedance-pH testing on acid-suppression medications has become a common method to evaluate patients with persistent GERD symptoms on medical therapy. If the pH component of the test shows normal esophageal acid exposure, the number of reflux events by impedance has been used to select patients that may benefit from antireflux surgery. However, most of these patients have not been confirmed to have GERD, and there is no clearly defined abnormal number of total reflux events by impedance-pH testing, on or off medications, that can reliably define patients with GERD.[24] Further, symptom indices are also not reliable for a diagnosis of GERD. It is recommended that patients with normal esophageal acid exposure on impedance-pH testing on medications undergo repeat pH testing off of their acid-suppression medications to confirm a diagnosis of GERD. Importantly, a firm diagnosis of GERD by pH testing is an important predicator of a good outcome with antireflux surgery. When combined with typical GERD symptoms and good response to acid-suppression medications, the presence of these 3 factors was associated with a good outcome in 97.4% of patients in a study analyzing factors predictive of outcome after Nissen fundoplication.[25] These factors remain useful and should be used in the selection of patients for antireflux surgery.

Surgical therapy has traditionally been reserved for patients with GERD symptoms that are partially or poorly responsive to medical therapy. Often these patients have late-stage GERD with large hiatal hernias and mucosal disease, including erosive esophagitis and Barrett's esophagus. Further, impaired esophageal motility is common in these patients. When confronted with advanced disease, it is a challenge for foregut surgeons to accomplish the goals of durable relief of GERD symptoms without inducing new symptoms or side effects with an antireflux procedure. In a sense it is similar to getting a dent in a new car versus in an old jalopy. The new car can be readily repaired to new car status, whereas the jalopy is unlikely to be anywhere near a new car after repair of the dent. The more damage to the esophagus before surgery the more difficult it is for antireflux surgery to be durable and not require adjunct techniques such as a Collis gastroplasty. Consequently, there is increasing support for the concept that patients with early reflux disease should be considered for antireflux surgery.[26]

What defines early reflux disease? At its simplest, early reflux disease is reflux that is confined to within the LES. Normally the LES occupies the entire abdominal esophagus and a portion of the lower thoracic esophagus, and is fully lined by squamous mucosa. In the absence of reflux-induced injury, the esophageal squamous mucosa directly abuts the acid-producing gastric oxyntic mucosa at the native GEJ but is protected by the functioning distal portion of the LES. Gastric distension with meals can lead to transient effacement of the distal abdominal portion of the LES and exposure of the acid-sensitive squamous mucosa to acidic gastric juice. This acid is present after meals in the acid pocket located near the GEJ.[27] Repetitive exposure of the distal esophageal squamous mucosa to acid produces inflammation, which over time can lead to a metaplastic change to cardiac epithelium. In early-stage GERD the GEJ and squamocolumnar junction are aligned and appear normal endoscopically, and therefore detection of metaplastic cardiac mucosa requires a biopsy at the GEJ.

Over time, repetitive episodes of gastric distension and exposure of the distal LES to acid not only damages the squamous mucosa but also leads to functional destruction of that portion of the LES. Gradually this process extends ever more proximally until LES competency is lost completely and gastric juice refluxes up into the esophagus. At this point the disease is no longer early and there is almost always cardiac mucosa present in the distal esophagus. The region between the normal squamous esophageal mucosa and the normal gastric oxyntic mucosa has been called the squamooxyntic gap, and the mucosa in this gap is always cardiac mucosa. The length of the gap, and correspondingly the length of cardiac mucosa, is related to the duration and severity of GERD.[28] The length of cardiac mucosa is also related to the risk of development of intestinal metaplasia. Once there is 3 cm of columnar-lined esophagus, intestinal metaplasia is almost always present.[29]

APPLICATION OF SURGICAL THERAPY TO PATIENTS WITH GASTROESOPHAGEAL REFLUX DISEASE

Given the spectrum of patients with GERD, surgeons offering antireflux therapy should be able to provide options tailored for that individual's disease state and expectations or desires in terms of the therapy. Highly symptomatic patients with a hiatal hernia, manometrically defective LES, and esophageal damage in the form of esophagitis or visible columnar-lined esophagus who are frustrated with their impaired quality of life from reflux disease and want optimal GERD therapy are particularly suited for a Nissen fundoplication. Patients with frustrating symptoms of GERD but no esophageal damage and an intact LES on manometry are candidates for a partial fundoplication, the LINX device, or an endoscopic fundoplication. The LINX device allows venting of the stomach with a belch and is associated with fewer side effects such as gas bloat, distension, and flatus than a Nissen fundoplication.[30] There is also evidence that a partial fundoplication is a good option in these patients, and, in a study comparing LINX with a Toupet partial fundoplication in patients with early reflux disease, Asti and colleagues[31] reported similar relief of GERD symptoms, improvement in quality of life, and satisfaction with the procedure with no difference in dysphagia, gas-related symptoms, or need for reoperation between groups. An important concept with the LINX is that, in order to maximize outcomes, any associated hiatal hernia must be repaired, and there is support by some investigators for complete hiatal dissection in all patients during LINX implantation.[2] Another option for patients with early disease is a TIF. This endoscopic fundoplication has been shown to have durable results in some patients, but it is clear again that any associated hiatal hernia needs to be repaired to achieve the best outcome.[32] This need has prompted combined laparoscopic repair of the hiatal hernia and TIF. However, there are minimal data comparing TIF with other partial fundoplications, such as the Toupet or anterior partial fundoplication, and, because neither of the alternative procedures requires instrumenting the esophagus, there is no justification for this approach outside of a trial at this time. The increased risk of esophageal injury with TIF has to be offset by some improvement in outcome with TIF compared with an alternative partial fundoplication done laparoscopically without the need to instrument the esophagus. At present, such data are lacking.

OUTCOME WITH A FUNDOPLICATION

Successful antireflux surgery is largely defined by 2 objectives: the achievement of long-term relief of reflux symptoms and the absence of side effects or complications from the operation. Both critically depend on establishing that the patient's symptoms are from GERD and that the optimal procedure for that patient is properly performed. Success can be expected in most patients if these criteria are met.

The advent of PPIs and laparoscopic fundoplication have changed the landscape of antireflux surgery. Before the introduction of the laparoscopic approach in the early 1990s, antireflux surgery was done as an open laparotomy or transthoracic procedure associated with significant morbidity, a typical hospital stay of 4 to 6 days, and a protracted recovery before the patient could return to full activities. The laparoscopic approach has changed all this dramatically. Most patients are back to routine activities within 1 to 2 weeks after surgery, the procedures are done as an outpatient or with an overnight stay, and morbidity has been substantially reduced.[33] Further, with the widespread use of PPIs, operating on patients with active esophagitis or strictures has become uncommon. This combination has led to antireflux surgery being adopted earlier in the course of reflux disease and in younger and healthier patients, leading to relief from typical GERD symptoms in more than 90% of patients in the short term in numerous studies.[34]

There have been several randomized trials comparing medical and surgical therapy. In the era before PPI medications, surgery was shown to be superior to medical therapy for control of GERD symptoms and complications.[35] In the modern era of PPI therapy, surgery has also been shown to be superior to medical therapy with omeprazole.[36] Another trial, named the LOTUS trial, compared esomeprazole with laparoscopic antireflux surgery. Dose adjustment of the esomeprazole was permitted, and at admission to the study all patients had symptoms that were well controlled on the medication. Again, antireflux surgery provided superior control of regurgitation symptoms compared with medical therapy.[37] Further, at 5 years of follow-up, 89% of antireflux surgery patients had normal esophageal acid exposure compared with 72% of patients in the medical arm who were tested while on their dose-adjusted esomeprazole medication.[38] The LOTUS trial also evaluated the presence and severity of symptoms in patients after antireflux surgery compared with those on medical therapy with esomeprazole. There was no difference in the severity of heartburn, epigastric pain, or diarrhea, but dysphagia, bloating, and flatulence remained more common in the antireflux group.[37] Long-term follow-up has shown that these symptoms are stable over time, and that dysphagia was uncommon in both groups, whereas flatulence was common in both groups.[39]

Longevity of Antireflux Surgery

One major criticism that has been leveled against laparoscopic antireflux surgery is that, although effective, it is not durable, and that most patients either need to go back on acid-suppression medications or have a redo operation. This concept is not supported by the available literature. Bernard Dallemagne was credited with doing the first laparoscopic Nissen fundoplication, Dallemagne and colleagues[40] reported on 100 consecutive patients followed for 10 years. Using a standardized symptom questionnaire, they found that reflux remained controlled after 10 years in 93% of patients after Nissen and 82% after Toupet fundoplication.[40] Likewise, in a report from Emory University with a mean follow-up of 11 years after surgery, heartburn and regurgitation symptoms were relieved in 90% of patients and 70% were off all reflux medications.[41] Csendes and colleagues[42] reported on 150 patients that had a laparoscopic Nissen fundoplication and were followed from 12 to 29 years postoperatively (mean of 15 years). Using a Visick scale, 119 patients (79%) were scored as I or II, meaning asymptomatic (101 patients) or mild/occasional reflux symptoms (18 patients). Further, on endoscopic follow-up, carditis had regressed to fundic mucosa in many patients. The investigators concluded that antireflux surgery was associated with long-lasting efficacy in most patients. Many patients are back on acid-suppression medications after antireflux surgery, but the reasons for this are varied, and typically not because the patient had objective evidence of recurrent reflux. A study evaluating this issue showed that, when patients back on acid-suppression medications after a fundoplication were evaluated with pH testing off their medications, more than 75% had normal esophageal acid exposure and did not need medications for reflux disease. However, PPI use is so common that patients are restarted on them for a variety of complaints, and I have seen patients back on PPIs after a total gastrectomy for cancer. Thus, resumption of PPI use is not a surrogate for a failed antireflux procedure.

ANTIREFLUX SURGERY AND BARRETT'S ESOPHAGUS

Patients with Barrett's esophagus typically have advanced reflux disease, which is logical because Barrett's esophagus develops in the setting of more advanced GERD, and these patients tend to have larger hiatal hernias, more impairment of LES function, and worse esophageal body function.[14] Consequently, it is not surprising that long-term results of antireflux surgery in patients with Barrett's esophagus tend to be inferior compared with the outcomes in patients with earlier stages of reflux disease. Hofstetter and colleagues[43] reported on 85 patients with Barrett's esophagus followed for a median of 5 years after antireflux surgery. Reflux symptoms were absent postoperatively in 79% of the patients. Postoperative 24-hour pH was normal in 17 of 21 patients (81%). A study from Australia followed 50 patients with Barrett's for a median of 11.9 years after fundoplication and reported that 86% had no or only mild reflux symptoms and 84% had normal acid exposure on Bravo 48-hour pH testing.[44] Although these results are good, they are about 10% lower than what would be expected in patients with earlier reflux disease and no Barrett's esophagus.

An important issue beyond the relief of symptoms with antireflux surgery in patients with Barrett's esophagus is the impact of the procedure on the metaplastic esophageal mucosa. In this area controversy still exists, but, over the last several decades, several publications have given credibility to the logical assumption that, if reflux causes Barrett's esophagus, and continued reflux drives Barrett's toward dysplasia and cancer, then stopping reflux with antireflux surgery should alter the natural history of the disease. At present there are data to show that antireflux surgery reduces the likelihood of intestinal metaplasia developing within cardiac mucosa, induces regression of intestinal metaplasia that is present before surgery, frequently leads to loss of low-grade dysplasia when present, and reduces the risk of progression of intestinal metaplasia to dysplasia and esophageal adenocarcinoma. Studies with gene expression have shown that, in part, these benefits of antireflux surgery are related to a reduction in the expression of inflammatory cytokines that seem to participate in Barrett's progression.[45–48]

Impact of Antireflux Surgery on the Development of Intestinal Metaplasia

Two studies have shown that antireflux surgery better protects against the development of intestinal metaplasia compared with medical therapy in patients with GERD. In a longitudinal prospective series of patients followed closely with endoscopic surveillance for a nonintestinalized columnar-lined esophagus, Oberg and colleagues[49] reported that, compared with patients on medical therapy, those that had an antireflux operation were 10.3 times less likely to develop intestinal metaplasia. Similarly, a study from Austria showed that, after 2 years of follow-up, 14.5% of patients on medical therapy developed Barrett's esophagus compared with no patient after antireflux surgery.[50] In the large German Pro-GERD (Progression of GERD) study, upper endoscopy in 3507 patients after medical GERD therapy for 2 years showed the development of Barrett's esophagus in 1.3%, but this was increased to 5.8% in patients with Los Angeles grade C or D esophagitis at entry into the study.[26] These studies confirm that medical therapy for GERD does not prevent the development of Barrett's esophagus, and raise concern that it may promote development of Barrett's rather than the more acid-related complications of reflux disease, such as esophagitis and stricture development. One explanation for the astounding increase in esophageal adenocarcinoma is that the current acid-suppression therapy for GERD is creating a large pool of patients with Barrett's esophagus, some of whom go on to then develop adenocarcinoma.

Impact of Antireflux Surgery on Intestinal Metaplasia Already Present Before Surgery

There are several studies that confirm that intestinal metaplasia can regress in length and in some patients be lost completely after antireflux surgery.[51–53] The likelihood of loss of intestinal metaplasia is related to the length of Barrett's esophagus, with shorter segments more likely to regress. Cardia intestinal metaplasia, sometimes called ultrashort Barrett's esophagus, was shown to regress to no intestinal metaplasia in 73% of patients after a fundoplication, whereas loss of intestinal metaplasia only occurred in 14% of patients with longer segments of Barrett's esophagus.[43,54] In a series by Low and colleagues,[55] 10 of 14 patients (71%) with Barrett's esophagus showed regression of the length, with 2 patients (14%) showing complete loss of intestinal metaplasia. Both of these patients had short-segment Barrett's esophagus. Similarly, Oelschlager and colleagues[56] reported complete loss of intestinal metaplasia after antireflux surgery in 30 of 54 patients (55%) with short-segment Barrett's esophagus but in none of 36 patients with long-segment Barrett's esophagus. In perhaps the largest series of carefully followed patients with short-segment Barrett's esophagus treated with laparoscopic Nissen fundoplication, Csendes and colleagues[57] reported loss of intestinal metaplasia in 61% of patients at a mean of 49 months. In addition, in a systematic review published in 2007, Chang and colleagues[52] reported a 17% overall rate of complete loss of intestinal metaplasia after antireflux surgery in patients with Barrett's esophagus. Recently, regression of intestinal metaplasia has also been shown to occur after LINX implantation, confirming the efficacy of this device to reduce esophageal acid exposure in appropriate candidates.[58]

Impact of Antireflux Surgery on Low-Grade Dysplasia

Antireflux surgery has also been show to induce regression of low-grade dysplasia.[51,52] Regression of low-grade to no dysplasia after a fundoplication has been reported by Hofstetter and colleagues[43] in 7 of 16 patients (44%) and by Oelschlager and colleagues[56] in 8 of 15 patients (53%). In the systematic review by Chang and colleagues,[52] antireflux surgery was associated with a 57% overall rate of regression of low-grade dysplasia. Most regression was to nondysplastic Barrett's esophagus, but in 4% regression was to no intestinal metaplasia. Although it could be argued that the diagnosis of low-grade dysplasia was not confirmed by a second pathologist and often represented inflammation rather than true low-grade dysplasia, any low-grade dysplasia is associated with an increased risk for progression, and regression should be considered a beneficial change for patients with Barrett's esophagus.[59]

Impact of Antireflux Surgery on Progression of Barrett's and Development of Esophageal Adenocarcinoma

In patients with Barrett's esophagus, several series have shown that, after antireflux surgery, progression to high-grade dysplasia or adenocarcinoma is rare.[43,55,60] In the systematic review by Chang and colleagues,[52] progression of any type was seen in only 4.2% of patients after antireflux surgery. Importantly, compared with continued medical therapy, several studies have shown a reduced risk of progression in patients treated with a fundoplication.[51] In a carefully followed group of patients with Barrett's esophagus, Oberg and colleagues[61] reported that the risk of developing low-grade dysplasia in patients on medical therapy was increased 2.3 times compared with those that had been treated with a fundoplication. Further, after fundoplication, no patient in that series progressed to high-grade dysplasia or adenocarcinoma. This difference was highly statistically significant compared with the frequency of progression to high-grade dysplasia or adenocarcinoma in medically treated patients.[61] To date there are limited data from randomized trials that report the risk of Barrett's esophagus progression in medically and surgically treated patients. A randomized trial from Spain limited to patients with Barrett's esophagus showed that, at a median follow-up of 6 years, patients with a functioning fundoplication were significantly less likely to have progressed to dysplasia compared with the medical treatment group.[62] In a subsequent analysis, the investigators reported that expression of Ki-67 and p53 remained stable over time in the group that had antireflux surgery but increased progressively and significantly in the medical therapy group.[63] These findings support the concept that antireflux surgery can induce a quiescent state in the Barrett's mucosa that may equate to a reduced likelihood of progression.

No discussion of the impact of antireflux surgery on Barrett's progression would be complete without including the series of studies published by Lagergren using Swedish population databases. Early studies from this group suggested antireflux surgery was not protective against the development of esophageal adenocarcinoma.[64] However, there were concerning methodologic flaws in this study.[65]

Subsequently, Lagergren and Viklund[66] showed that a failed fundoplication is a risk factor for Barrett's progression, and conversely a functioning fundoplication may reduce the risk of progression.[67,68]

Antireflux Surgery in Patients with Barrett's: A Word of Caution

Barrett's esophagus represents long-standing reflux disease because it is estimated to take 5 or more years for Barrett's esophagus to develop.[51] Longer segments of Barrett's esophagus are associated with more physiologic abnormalities, including larger hiatal hernias and worse LES function.[69] These anatomic and functional abnormalities make successful treatment of patients with long-segment Barrett's more difficult with both PPIs and antireflux surgery. Given that the frequency of a recurrent hiatal hernia or failure of the fundoplication is increased in patients with Barrett's esophagus, particular attention must be paid to securely closing the crura and addressing tension in these patients to minimize the risk of recurrent GERD. When a short esophagus is encountered, a Collis gastroplasty should be considered. However, a Collis gastroplasty can be problematic in patients with Barrett's esophagus, particularly if ablation becomes necessary, and so in some patients with Barrett's esophagus a nonoperative approach may be warranted. If an operation is undertaken, every effort must be made to prevent failure of the fundoplication given the evidence presented earlier that a failed fundoplication is a risk factor for progression of Barrett's esophagus to adenocarcinoma. Given the complexity of patients with Barrett's esophagus and the implications of a failed operation, only high-volume foregut surgeons expert in the management of Barrett's esophagus should evaluate and operate on these patients.

SUMMARY

Antireflux surgery is challenging, and has become even more challenging with the introduction of alternative endoscopic and laparoscopic options for patients with GERD. The Nissen fundoplication has stood the test of time and has evolved from open laparotomy or thoracotomy to a minimally invasive laparoscopic approach with a short hospital stay, rapid return to normal activities, and minimal perioperative morbidity. It remains the gold standard for the durable relief of GERD symptoms and esophagitis. However, the degree of the fundoplication can be tailored and, in patients with early reflux disease, such as those with heartburn or regurgitation symptoms without esophageal damage, a partial fundoplication offers fewer side effects and may be the preferred approach. Alternatively, the LINX device or an endoscopic antireflux procedure may be ideal in patients with little or no hiatal hernia and early reflux disease. All antireflux procedures have a failure rate, and it is important to understand factors that are associated with failure and minimize them to ensure optimal outcomes in patients that present for antireflux surgery. A failed antireflux procedure is troublesome for the patient, can lead to worse reflux disease than the patient had before the procedure, and is a risk factor for progression in patients with Barrett's esophagus. Consequently, the selection of patients for antireflux surgery as well as the choice of the procedure, be it a fundoplication, the LINX device, or an endoscopic approach, requires a thorough understanding of esophageal physiology and the pros and cons of various options. It is best done by focused foregut surgeons that maintain a high volume of procedures and can offer all available options to patients with GERD and guide patients to the best procedure for their disease stage and expectations.

DISCLOSURE

None.

REFERENCES

1. Bowrey D, Peters J. Laparoscopic Esophageal Surgery. Surg Clin North Am 2000;80:12131242.
2. Tatum J, et al. Minimal versus obligatory dissection of the diaphragmatic hiatus during magnetic sphincter augmentation surgery. Surg Endosc 2019;33:782–8.
3. Janu P, et al. Laparoscopic hiatal hernia repair followed by transoral incisionless fundoplication with EsophyX device: efficacy and safety in two community hospitals. Surg Innov 2019;26(6):675–86.
4. Collis JL. An operation for hiatus hernia with short esophagus. J Thorac Surg 1957;34:768–78.
5. Zehetner J, et al. Laparoscopic versus open repair of paraesophageal hernia: the second decade. J Am Coll Surg 2011;212(5):813–20.
6. Allison PR. Reflux esophagitis, sliding hiatal hernia, and the anatomy of repair. Surg Gynecol Obstet 1951;92(4):419–31.
7. Allison PR. Hiatus hernia: (a 20-year retrospective survey). Ann Surg 1973;178(3): 273–6.
8. Muller-Stich B, et al. Repair of paraesophageal hiatal hernias-is a fundoplication needed? A randomized controlled pilot trial. J Am Coll Surg 2015;221:602–10.
9. Oleynikov D, et al. Total fundoplication is the operation of choice for patients with gastroesophageal reflux and defective peristalsis. Surg Endosc 2002;16(6): 909–13.
10. Patti MG, et al. Total fundoplication is superior to partial fundoplication even when esophageal peristalsis is weak.[see comment]. J Am Coll Surg 2004;198(6): 863–9 [discussion: 869–70].
11. Zhu ZJ, Chen LQ, Duranceau A. Long-term results of total versus partial fundoplication following esophagomyotomy for primary esophageal motor disorders. World J Surg 2008;32:401–7.
12. Ayazi S, et al. Clinical significance of esophageal outflow resistance imposed by a Nissen fundoplication. J Am Coll Surg 2019;229:210–6.
13. Horvath KD, et al. Laparoscopic Toupet fundoplication is an inadequate procedure for patients with severe reflux disease. J Gastrointest Surg 1999;3(6):583–91.
14. Lord RVN, et al. Hiatal hernia, lower esophageal sphincter incompetence, and effectiveness of Nissen fundoplication in the spectrum of gastroesophageal reflux disease. J Gastrointest Surg 2009;13(4):602–10.
15. Hinder RA, et al. Relationship of a satisfactory outcome to normalization of delayed gastric emptying after Nissen fundoplication. Ann Surg 1989;210(4): 458–64 [discussion: 464–5].
16. Lundell L, et al. Comparing laparoscopic antireflux surgery with esomeprazole in the management of patients with chronic gastro-oesophageal reflux disease: a 3-year interim analysis of the LOTUS trial. Gut 2008;57(9):1207–13.
17. Lundell L, et al. Seven-year follow-up of a randomized clinical trial comparing proton-pump inhibition with surgical therapy for reflux esophagitis. Br J Surg 2007;94:198–203.
18. Broeders JA, et al. Reflux and belching after 270 degree versus 360 degree laparoscopic posterior fundoplication. Ann Surg 2012;255(1):59–65.
19. Cai W, et al. Ten-year clinical outcome of a prospective randomized clinical trial of laparoscopic Nissen versus anterior 180(degrees) partial fundoplication. Br J Surg 2008;95(12):1501–5.
20. Falkenback D, et al. Is the course of gastroesophageal reflux disease progressive? A 21-year follow-up. Scand J Gastroenterol 2009;44(11):1277–87.

21. Finks JF, Wei Y, Birkmeyer JD. The rise and fall of antireflux surgery in the United States. Surg Endosc 2006;20:1698–701.
22. Malfertheiner P, et al. Evolution of gastro-oesophageal reflux disease over 5 years under routine medical care–the ProGERD study. Aliment Pharmacol Ther 2012; 35(1):154–64.
23. Schwameis K, et al. Is pH testing necessary before antireflux surgery in patients with endoscopic erosive esophagitis. J Gastrointest Surg 2018;22:8–12.
24. Ward MA, et al. Can impedance-pH testing on medications reliably identify patients with GERD as defined by pathologic esophageal acid exposure of medications? J Gastrointest Surg 2019;23:1301–8.
25. Campos GM, et al. Multivariate analysis of factors predicting outcome after laparoscopic Nissen fundoplication. J Gastrointest Surg 1999;3(3):292–300.
26. Labenz J, et al. Prospective follow-up data from the ProGERD study suggest that GERD is not a categorial disease.[see comment]. Am J Gastroenterol 2006; 101(11):2457–62.
27. Mitchell DR, et al. The role of the acid pocket in gastroesophageal disease. J Clin Gastroenterol 2016;50:111–9.
28. Chandrasoma P, et al. The histologic squamo-oxyntic gap: an accurate and reproducible diagnostic marker of gastroesophageal reflux disease. Am J Surg Pathol 2010;34(11):1574–81.
29. Chandrasoma PT, et al. Distribution and significance of epithelial types in columnar-lined esophagus. Am J Surg Pathol 2001;25(9):1188–93.
30. Reynolds JL, et al. Magnetic sphincter augmentation with the LINX device for gastroesophageal reflux disease after U.S. Food and Drug Administration approval. Am Surg 2014;80(10):1034–8.
31. Asti E, et al. Longitudinal comparison of quality of life in patients undergoing laparoscopic Toupet fundoplication versus magnetic sphincter augmentation. Medicine 2016;95:1–6.
32. Min MX, Ganz RA. Update in procedural therapy for GERD–magnetic sphincter augmentation, endoscopic transoral incisionless fundoplication vs laparoscopic Nissen fundoplication. Curr Gastroenterol Rep 2014;16(2):374.
33. Schlottmann F, Strassle PD, Patti M. Surgery for benign esophageal disorders in the US: risk factors for complications and trends in morbidity. Surg Endosc 2018; 32:3675–862.
34. Bowrey DJ, Peters JH. Laparoscopic esophageal surgery. Surg Clin North Am 2000;80(4):1213–42, vii.
35. Spechler SJ. Comparison of medical and surgical therapy for complicated gastroesophageal reflux disease in veterans. N Engl J Med 1992;326:786–92.
36. Lundell L, et al. Continued (5 years) follow-up of a randomised clinical study comparing anti-reflux surgery and omeprazole in gastroesophageal reflux surgery. Gastroenterology 2000;118(4):A191.
37. Galmiche J-P, et al. Laparoscopic antireflux surgery vs esomeprazole treatment for chronic GERD: the LOTUS randomized clinical trial. JAMA 2011;305(19): 1969–77.
38. Hatlebakk JG, et al. Gastroesophageal acid reflux control 5 years after antireflux surgery compared with long-term esomeprazole therapy. Clin Gastroenterol Hepatol 2016;14:678–85.
39. Lundell L, et al. Comparison of outcomes twelve years after antireflux surgery or omeprazole maintenance therapy for reflux esophagitis. Clin Gastroenterol Hepatol 2009;7(12):1292–8 [quiz: 1260].

40. Dallemagne B, et al. Clinical results of laparoscopic fundoplication at ten years after surgery. Surg Endosc 2006;20:159–65.

41. Morgenthal CB, et al. The durability of laparoscopic Nissen fundoplication: 11-year outcomes. J Gastrointest Surg 2007;11:693–700.

42. Csendes A, et al. Long-term (15 year) objective evaluation of 150 patients after laparoscopic Nissen fundoplication. Surgery 2019;166(5):886–94.

43. Hofstetter WL, et al. Long-term outcome of antireflux surgery in patients with Barrett's esophagus. Ann Surg 2001;234(4):532–8 [discussion: 538–9].

44. Knight BC, et al. Long-term efficacy of laparoscopic antireflux surgery on regression of Barrett's esophagus using Bravo wireless pH monitoring. Ann Surg 2017;266:1000–5.

45. Shimizu D, et al. Increasing cyclooxygenase-2 (cox-2) gene expression in the progression of Barrett's esophagus to adenocarcinoma correlates with that of Bcl-2. Int J Cancer 2006;119(4):765–70.

46. Vallbohmer D, et al. Cdx-2 expression in squamous and metaplastic columnar epithelia of the esophagus. Dis Esophagus 2006;19(4):260–6.

47. Vallbohmer D, et al. Antireflux surgery normalizes cyclooxygenase-2 expression in squamous epithelium of the distal esophagus. Am J Gastroenterol 2006;101(7):1458–66.

48. Oh DS, et al. Reduction of interleukin 8 gene expression in reflux esophagitis and Barrett's esophagus with antireflux surgery. Arch Surg 2007;142(6):554–9 [discussion: 559–60].

49. Oberg S, et al. Endoscopic surveillance of columnar-lined esophagus: frequency of intestinal metaplasia detection and impact of antireflux surgery. Ann Surg 2001;234(5):619–26.

50. Wetscher GJ, et al. Efficacy of medical therapy and antireflux surgery to prevent Barrett's metaplasia in patients with gastroesophageal reflux disease. Ann Surg 2001;234(5):627–32.

51. DeMeester SR, DeMeester TR. Columnar Mucosa and Intestinal Metaplasia of the Esophagus: Fifty Years of Controversy. Ann Surg 2000;231(3):303–21.

52. Chang EY, et al. The effect of antireflux surgery on esophageal carcinogenesis in patients with barrett esophagus: a systematic review. Ann Surg 2007;246(1):11–21.

53. Morrow E, et al. The impact of laparoscopic anti-reflux surgery in patients with Barrett's esophagus. Surg Endosc 2014;28(12):3279–84.

54. DeMeester SR, et al. The impact of an antireflux procedure on intestinal metaplasia of the cardia. Ann Surg 1998;228(4):547–56.

55. Low DE, et al. Histological and anatomic changes in Barrett's esophagus after antireflux surgery. Am J Gastroenterol 1999;94(1):80–5.

56. Oelschlager BK, et al. Clinical and pathologic response of Barrett's esophagus to laparoscopic antireflux surgery. Ann Surg 2003;238(4):458–64 [discussion: 464–6].

57. Csendes A, et al. Late results of the surgical treatment of 125 patients with short-segment Barrett esophagus. Arch Surg 2009;144(10):921–7.

58. Alicuben ET, et al. Regression of intestinal metaplasia following magnetic sphincter augmentation device placement. Surg Endosc 2019;33:576–9.

59. Solansky D, et al. Barrett Esophagus length, nodularity, and low-grade dysplasia are predictive of progression to esophageal adenocarcinoma. J Clin Gastroenterol 2019;53:361–5.

60. McDonald ML, et al. Barrett's esophagus: does an antireflux procedure reduce the need for endoscopic surveillance? J Thorac Cardiovasc Surg 1996;111(6): 1135–8 [discussion: 1139–40].
61. Oberg S, et al. Barrett esophagus: risk factors for progression to dysplasia and adenocarcinoma. Ann Surg 2005;242(1):49–54.
62. Parrilla P, et al. Long-term results of a randomized prospective study comparing medical and surgical treatment of Barrett's esophagus.[see comment]. Ann Surg 2003;237(3):291–8.
63. Martinez de Haro LF, et al. Long-term follow-up of malignancy biomarkers in patients with Barrett's esophagus undergoing medical or surgical treatment. Ann Surg 2012;255(5):916–21.
64. Lagergren J, et al. The risk of esophageal adenocarcinoma after antireflux surgery. Gastroenterology 2010;138(4):1297–301.
65. DeMeester SR. Antireflux surgery and the risk of esophageal adenocarcinoma: an antithetical view of the data from sweden. Ann Surg 2013;257(4):583–5.
66. Lagergren J, Viklund P. Is esophageal adenocarcinoma occurring late after antireflux surgery due to persistent postoperative reflux?[see comment]. World J Surg 2007;31(3):465–9.
67. Lofdahl HE, et al. Risk factors for esophageal adenocarcinoma after antireflux surgery. Ann Surg 2013;257:579–82.
68. Maret-Ouda J, et al. Antireflux surgery and risk of esophageal adenocarcinoma: a systemic review and meta-analysis. Ann Surg 2016;2016:251–7.
69. Oberg S, et al. The extent of Barrett's esophagus depends on the status of the lower esophageal sphincter and the degree of esophageal acid exposure. J Thorac Cardiovasc Surg 1999;117(3):572–80.

Magnetic Sphincter Augmentation for Gastroesophageal Reflux Disease

Colin Dunn, MD[a,1], Nikolai Bildzukewicz, MD[b],
John Lipham, MD[c,*]

KEYWORDS

- Magnetic sphincter augmentation • Gastroesophageal reflux disease • Hiatal hernia
- Fundoplication

KEY POINTS

- Magnetic sphincter augmentation with LINX is an effective surgical treatment of reflux disease.
- Intermediate-term outcomes have shown safety and efficacy of the LINX device compared with both laparoscopic fundoplication and medical therapy.
- New research has expanded on indications for magnetic sphincter augmentation, including after failure of single proton pump inhibitor therapy rather than twice-daily therapy, in patients with Barrett's esophagus, and in patients with large hiatal hernias.

 Video content accompanies this article at http://www.giendo.theclinics.com.

INTRODUCTION

Gastroesophageal reflux disease (GERD) has an estimated prevalence of 18.1% to 27.8% in North America and leads to estimated costs of US$9 to 12 billion annually.[1,2] The prevalence of GERD has been steadily increasing with time.[1] One-third of patients taking a daily proton pump inhibitor (PPI) for GERD report incomplete resolution of their symptoms.[3] In such cases, it is common to double the dosage of PPI to twice daily.[4] However, up to 60% of patients who do not respond to PPIs may have nonacid reflux disease.[4] In this disorder, the symptoms arise from refluxate that is

[a] General Surgery Rutgers NJMS, 185 South Orange Avenue, Medical Science Building, Room G 594, Newark, NJ 07101, USA; [b] The Advanced GI/MIS Fellowship, Keck Medical Center of USC, 1510 San Pablo Street, HCC I, Suite 514, Los Angeles, CA 90033-4612, USA; [c] Upper GI Cancer, Keck Medical Center of USC, 1510 San Pablo Street, HCC I, Suite 514, Los Angeles, CA 90033-4612, USA
[1] Present address: 1510 San Pablo Street, HCC I, Suite 514, Los Angeles, CA 90033-4612.
* Corresponding author.
E-mail address: john.lipham@med.usc.edu

Gastrointest Endoscopy Clin N Am 30 (2020) 325–342
https://doi.org/10.1016/j.giec.2019.12.010
1052-5157/20/© 2020 Elsevier Inc. All rights reserved.

giendo.theclinics.com

neutral in pH, and, as such, these patients do not respond to PPIs. Gastric fundoplication is the traditional surgical method of treating esophageal reflux, with initial success rates greater than 90% at high-volume centers. However, fundoplication is technically difficult, requires an overnight or inpatient stay, and is associated with gas bloat syndrome. In addition, impaired belching and vomiting with subsequent feeling of distention is present in up to 25% of patients with traditional fundoplication.[5,6] Recurrence is also a concern, with average 10-year recurrence rates of 10% to 15%.[7] Magnetic sphincter augmentation (MSA) is a newer surgical option to treat reflux disease that attempts to mitigate these issues. This article focuses on evaluating patients for MSA with the LINX device, implanting the device, and managing the patients postoperatively. This article discusses short-term and long-term outcomes, as well as associated complications, controversies, and future research directions.

ADVENT OF LINX

For those patients who do not respond to a twice-daily dose of PPI or do not want to take PPIs for life, laparoscopic fundoplication is the traditional recommendation. Because of the aforementioned side effects of this procedure, as few as 1% of eligible patients with GERD opt for this surgery.[8] However, 40% of patients with GERD are symptomatic despite PPI therapy, resulting in a treatment gap. Many patients have GERD symptoms that are refractory to PPI, but these symptoms are not severe enough for them to seek surgical intervention.[9] In addition, outcomes with fundoplication are highly variable in the surgical community. The best outcomes are seen at high-volume specialized centers.[10] To fill this treatment gap, a new solution was necessary, one that was as effective as the fundoplication but with minimal side effects and that was less technically demanding on the surgeon.

MSA was created as a response to the treatment gap in the mid to late 2000s. The LINX device is made up of interconnected rare earth magnets, each of which is encased in a titanium bead, forming a ring (like a bracelet) when placed circumferentially around the esophagus near the gastroesophageal junction (**Fig. 1**). The device is

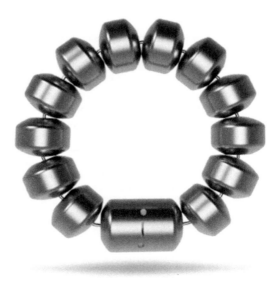

Fig. 1. The LINX device. (© Ethicon, Inc. Reproduced with permission.)

noncompressive, and the strength of the magnets is precisely calibrated to restore lower esophageal sphincter (LES) function while preserving normal physiologic function. At rest, the magnetic force holds the beads close together to prevent reflux from occurring (**Fig. 2**).[11] The magnetic beads separate in response to a food bolus, then resume their original configuration (see **Fig. 2**).[11]

The LINX device allows normal physiologic function, generating about 20 mm Hg of resistance at the gastroesophageal junction.[12] Normal peristaltic pressures during a swallow range from 35 to 80 mm Hg, which generates enough pressure for the food bolus to overcome the resistance of the magnets. Normal intragastric pressure ranges from 5 to 10 mm Hg, which allows the higher resistance of the magnets to minimize reflux. However, if the patients need to belch or vomit, they can increase their intragastric pressure to overcome the resistance of the magnets.

The procedure is also technically simpler than a fundoplication. It is minimally invasive, takes less than an hour to perform, and most patients are discharged on the same day of the procedure. For these reasons, MSA with the LINX device is an attractive alternative for antireflux surgery. The LINX device does have 1 contraindication (allergy to titanium, nickel). There are also precautions, most of which are related to having no additional gastroesophageal disorder before surgery (**Box 1**).

DIAGNOSIS

Evaluating a patient for MSA is no different than the standard work-up for any patient with GERD. This process begins with a history and physical. Patients usually describe retrosternal burning in the postprandial period. Other symptoms include dysphagia, chest pain, chronic cough, hoarseness, or wheezing.[13] Complaints of dysphagia can also indicate a stricture or dysmotility; this requires careful attention. A response to PPIs does not definitely establish the diagnosis of GERD, although it does help identify patients who would do well following antireflux surgery.[14]

If uncomplicated GERD is diagnosed, the patient begins treatment with a PPI.[15] If alarming symptoms are present, the patient undergoes an esophagogastroduodenoscopy with potential biopsy of any areas suspicious for metaplasia or dysplasia.[15] Irregular linear ulcerations visualized in the distal esophagus are consistent with

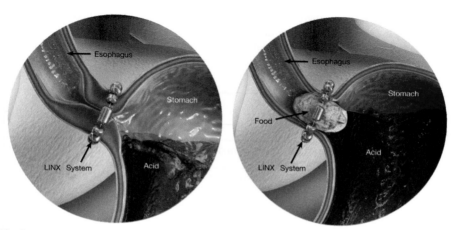

Fig. 2. Functioning LINX device. The device maintains competency of the LES but dilates to allow passage of a food bolus. (© Ethicon, Inc. Reproduced with permission.)

Box 1
LINX precautions
Existing esophageal motility disorder
Esophageal or gastric cancer
Intra-abdominal infection or perforation
Allergy to titanium or nickel
Presence of electrical implant
Patient requiring MRI greater than 1.5 T
Los Angeles classification C or D esophagitis
Barrett's
Esophageal or gastric varices or strictures
Body mass index greater than 35
Scleroderma
Pregnant women
Age less than 21 years
Preoperative dysphagia more than once a week for past 3 months

esophagitis, and this is graded using the Los Angeles classification on a scale of increasing severity from A to D (**Table 1**).[16] The gastroesophageal junction (GEJ) is closely examined for the presence of a hiatal hernia and the Hill grade (I–IV) of the valve is also noted.[17]

A pH study is still the gold standard for diagnosing GERD, and our patients undergo 48 hours (and even up to 96 hours) of ambulatory esophageal pH monitoring. This monitoring is usually performed with the patients off PPIs for at least 7 days before the study. Ambulatory pH monitoring is conducted by attaching a pH sensor to the distal esophagus at the time of endoscopy. If during the endoscopy, LA class C or D esophagitis is present, this testing can generally be deferred.[18]

To evaluate esophageal motility, a thorough videoesophagram (VEG) is performed. If any significant dysmotility is noted on this study, high-resolution esophageal manometry is conducted to better define the dysmotility. Our group recently published findings that a normal VEG can obviate routine esophageal manometry.[19] Out of 418 patients undergoing VEG and esophageal manometry before antireflux surgery, 231

Table 1		
Los Angeles esophagitis classification		
Grade	**Description**	
A	One (or more) mucosal breaks no longer than 5 mm, which do not extend between the tops of 2 mucosal folds	
B	One (or more) mucosal breaks more than 5 mm long, which do not extend between the tops of 2 mucosal folds	
C	One (or more) mucosal breaks that are continuous between the tops of 2 or more mucosal folds but that involve <75% of the circumference	
D	One (or more) mucosal breaks that involve at least 75% of the esophageal circumference	

Table 2	
Barrett's esophagus classification	
Segment Length	**Description**
Short	Squamocolumnar junction ≥1 cm above the gastroesophageal junction
Long	Squamocolumnar junction ≥3 cm above the gastroesophageal junction

patients had a normal VEG. Of these patients, only 1 had abnormal motility, resulting in a sensitivity of 96.4%.[19]

During the initial clinical trials, the ideal candidate for MSA had mild to moderate symptoms, no or small (<3 cm) hiatal hernia, a pathologic amount of reflux on pH testing, and normal esophageal motility. With additional clinical experience and research, the criteria have been expanded to include patients with larger hiatal hernias, Barrett's esophagus (**Table 2**), and mild dysmotility.

TECHNIQUE OF IMPLANTATION

Following induction of general anesthesia, the patient is placed in a modified lithotomy position with the arms tucked at the sides. The table is then placed in a steep reverse Trendelenburg position. The patient's abdomen is accessed in the left upper quadrant just a few centimeters cephalad and lateral to the umbilicus using a 5-mm Optiview trocar. Pneumoperitoneum is established at a pressure of 15 mm Hg of carbon dioxide. An 8-mm trocar is then placed in the left upper quadrant in the midclavicular line in a subcostal position. A 5-mm trocar is placed in the far left upper quadrant in the left anterior axillary line. A final 5-mm trocar is placed in the right upper quadrant in a subcostal position. A Nathanson liver retractor is placed in the subxiphoid position and used to elevate the left lobe of the liver.

Attention is then directed toward the diaphragmatic hiatus, assessing for the presence or absence of a hiatal hernia (Video 1). The stomach is retracted to the left. Dissection begins at the pars flaccida of the gastrohepatic ligament (**Fig. 3**).

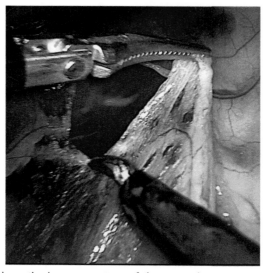

Fig. 3. Dissection along the lesser curvature of the stomach.

Electrocautery is used to continue the dissection up toward the right crus, carefully inspecting for a replaced or accessory left hepatic vessel. On reaching the right crus, it is scored using electrocautery and blunt dissection is used to establish a plane between the right crus and the esophagus and/or hernia sac (**Fig. 4**). This dissection is then continued anteriorly over the esophagus in a circumferential fashion toward the left crus. Once reached, the left crus is scored in a similar fashion and blunt dissection is continued to mobilize the esophagus laterally and posteriorly (**Fig. 5**). If present, the hernia sac is circumferentially mobilized out of the lower mediastinum and reduced into the abdominal cavity. A 6-mm (0.25-inch) Penrose drain is introduced through a retroesophageal window, then wrapped around the esophagus (**Fig. 6**). Grasping this Penrose drain aids in retraction. The distal esophagus is then circumferentially mobilized out of the lower mediastinum to ensure an adequate intra-abdominal length of approximately 2 to 3 cm. The patient's hiatus is then reapproximated using multiple interrupted sutures of 0-Ethibond thrown in a figure-of-eight fashion and secured using the Ti-KNOT device (**Fig. 7**). Care is taken to not encroach on the esophagus too tightly. Following hiatal closure, the Penrose drain is grasped and placed on traction, and the posterior vagus nerve is then gently dissected off the distal esophagus at the level of the GEJ (**Fig. 8**). The Penrose drain is then reintroduced through this window and laid open posteriorly (not grasped). The LINX sizing tool is then introduced through the right upper quadrant trocar and advanced over the Penrose drain through the retroesophageal window. The sizing tool is then deployed anteriorly over the esophagus until the magnet engages with the metal band on the distal shaft (**Fig. 9**) to form a loop around the esophagus. The plunger on the sizing tool is gently pulled back 1 click at a time, tightening the loop. This process continues until the loop rests comfortably on the distal esophagus without impinging it. Once achieved, the handle of the sizing tool is visualized and a green mark indicates the size of the LINX device. The plunger is further advanced, and the sizing tool should start to constrict the esophagus at the

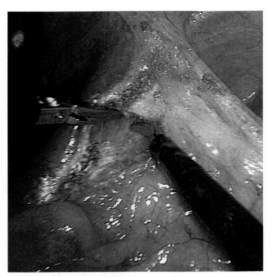

Fig. 4. Dissection of the right crus. (*From* Lipham JC, Taiganides PA, Louie BE, Ganz RA, Demeester TR. Safety analysis of first 1000 patients treated with magnetic sphincter augmentation for gastroesophageal reflux disease. Diseases of the Esophagus 2015;28 (4):305-11; with permission.)

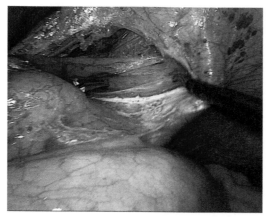

Fig. 5. Dissection of the left crus.

next click. This process continues until the tension on the loop is great enough, causing it to pop or separate. This pop should occur at 3 sizes smaller than the size chosen based on the visual cues as described earlier. This second step is a quality-assurance measure. If there is ever a discrepancy, the greater size is chosen. The entire process of sizing is generally repeated 2 to 3 times.

The appropriately sized LINX device is opened onto the field in a sterile fashion and introduced into the peritoneal cavity. A laparoscopic grasper or empty needle driver is placed through the retroesophageal window (anterior to the posterior vagus nerve) from medial to lateral. One of the 2 sutures on the LINX device is then handed to the grasper and the LINX device is gently guided through this tunnel from lateral to medial (**Fig. 10**). The 2 ends of the LINX device are brought together anteriorly over the esophagus and the magnetic clasp of the device is securely engaged. Close inspection of the clasp reveals only 1 window between the 2 beads and the device remains seated when both sutures are pulled 180° in opposite directions. Both sutures are cut and are removed along with the Penrose drain. A final inspection of the LINX device is performed (**Fig. 11**). If satisfactory, the liver retractor and trocars are

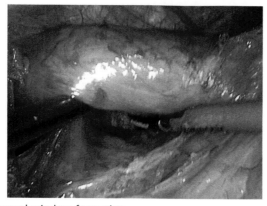

Fig. 6. Retroesophageal window formation.

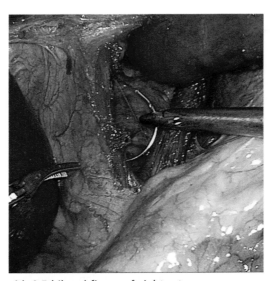

Fig. 7. Cruroplasty with 0-Ethibond figure-of-eight sutures.

removed under direct visualization while simultaneously desufflating the abdomen. Skin incisions are closed using buried interrupted sutures of 4-0 Monocryl and Dermabond is applied as a dressing.

POSTOPERATIVE CARE

The patient is usually discharged home the day of the procedure. A soft diet is initiated immediately following the procedure, and the patient is instructed to resume a normal diet within a few days. Importantly, the patient is encouraged to snack frequently (every 2–3 hours while awake) for the first few weeks to help minimize postoperative dysphagia. If any significant dysphagia develops, a short course of oral steroids is prescribed. For persistent dysphagia, endoscopic pneumatic dilation is delayed until 3 to 4 months after surgery, because outcomes have not improved with earlier intervention and this can worsen dysphagia.[20]

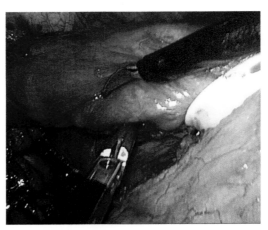

Fig. 8. Dissection of posterior vagal trunk.

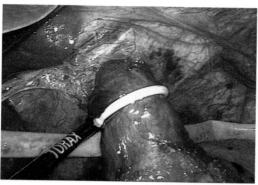

Fig. 9. Deployment of the sizing tool.

CLINICAL DATA FOR MAGNETIC SPHINCTER AUGMENTATION

In 2008, the first feasibility trial of the LINX device was published.[21] Forty-one patients were studied. At 3 months after implantation, 89% of patients were no longer taking their PPIs. The median GERD Health Related Quality of Life (GERD-HRQL) score also decreased to 2.6 from 26 at 6 months postoperatively, showing that the patients had a statistically and clinically significant improvement in their quality of life. Mild dysphagia occurred in 45% of patients. All of this resolved without intervention, except for 1 patient with persistent dysphagia who required device removal 8 months after surgery. Furthermore, all patients had normal manometry results at 3 months after surgery.

Because of these encouraging results, researchers continued to follow this cohort of patients. A follow-up study was published in 2010.[22] At 2 years, the GERD-HRQL was 2.4 and 86% of patients remained off of PPIs. In addition, this cohort was followed up to 4 years with 80% of patients still off their PPIs and 100% of the patients continuing to report improved GERD-related quality of life.[23] Only 3 devices were removed during that time period.

For further validation, a larger, prospective, nonrandomized study was conducted between 13 centers in the United States and 1 in the Netherlands and was published

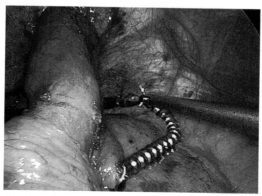

Fig. 10. Positioning the LINX device posterior to the esophagus and anterior to the posterior vagal trunk. (© Ethicon, Inc. Reproduced with permission.)

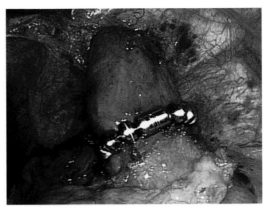

Fig. 11. Final correct positioning of the LINX device. (© Ethicon, Inc. Reproduced with permission.)

by Ganz and colleagues.[24] One hundred patients underwent the MSA procedure. The primary end point was either normalized distal esophageal acid exposure during 24-hour pH monitoring or a 50% reduction in the total time in which the pH was less than 4, compared with baseline measurements. The end points were recorded at 1 year postoperatively. At the 1 -week, 3-weeks, 6-months, and annual postoperative visits, researchers assessed the quality of life with the GERD-HRQL score as well as the use/dose of PPIs. The primary end point was achieved in 64% of patients. PPI use declined to 14% at the 1-year mark and remained low at 13% at 3 years after device implantation. Three years after the surgery, 94% of patients were overall satisfied with the procedure. There were 4 patients who required device removal. Nineteen patients had endoscopic dilatation procedures for persistent dysphagia.

Based on the results of this landmark study, the device was approved for use by the US Food and Drug Administration.[5] However, detractors pointed out that a primary end point achievement of only 64% was low, and that 4 device removals suggested the device was potentially unsafe. Follow-up results at 5 years showed no additional adverse outcomes or safety concerns, and significant clinical improvement because 83% of the patients met the primary end point.[5]

Concurrently, another prospective cohort study was conducted at a single institution in Italy.[25] One hundred consecutive patients underwent MSA. The study cohort included expanded inclusion criteria, accepting patients who had received radiofrequency ablation for short-segment Barrett's esophagus, or patients with hiatal hernias up to 4 cm.[25] A greater than 50% reduction in GERD-HRQL scores was seen in 93% of patients. Eighty-five percent of patients discontinued their PPIs. The median DeMeester score was reduced to 11.3 from 30.1. Three devices were removed during the study period, 2 for persistent dysphagia and 1 for failure to resolve reflux symptoms. Only 2 patients required endoscopic dilatation for persistent dysphagia.

MAGNETIC SPHINCTER AUGMENTATION VERSUS FUNDOPLICATION

Although prospective cohort studies were informative, a comparison against laparoscopic fundoplication (LF) was necessary. In 2015, Reynolds and colleagues[26] used propensity score matching on 9 factors associated with GERD to simulate a randomized controlled trial comparing 50 MSA patients with 50 patients who received a laparoscopic Nissen fundoplication (LNF). There were no differences in GERD-HRQL or

PPI use at 1 year after surgery. Dysphagia was also not significantly different between the 2 groups. A significantly greater percentage of patients could successfully belch or vomit in the MSA group compared with the fundoplication group (belch 91.5% vs 74.5%, $P = .028$; vomit 95.7% vs 78.7%, $P = .004$).

Several other prospective studies were done, showing similar results highlighting the comparative safety and efficacy of MSA compared with LF.[27–30] Each of these studies found comparable relief of GERD-related symptoms with preserved ability to belch and vomit with MSA, but not with LF. Riegler and colleagues[27] found a lower level of reoperation for MSA compared with LNF (4.0% vs 6.4%) and a greater reduction in severe GERD symptoms with MSA (55% vs 47%). MSA was also compared with laparoscopic Toupet fundoplication to further characterize its efficacy.[31] Asti and colleagues[31] compared 238 consecutive patients undergoing either Toupet fundoplication or MSA, with 100% of the cohort being evaluated at 1 year postoperatively. The 2 groups underwent propensity score matching on the presence of esophagitis, Barrett's esophagus, hiatal hernia size, Hill grade, and body mass index (BMI).[31] There was no difference found between the 2 groups when comparing GERD-HRQL, PPI use, gas-related symptoms, dysphagia, and need for reoperation.[31]

In 2018, a systematic review and meta-analysis was done to compare MSA with LF.[32] Seven separate studies were pooled to create a cohort of 1211 patients, 686 in the MSA group and 524 in the LF group. There were no differences in GERD-HRQL. The ability to belch and vomit had a pooled hazard ratio of 10.10 for MSA versus fundoplication (95% confidence interval, 5.33–19.15; $P<.001$). There was a trend toward increased postoperative dysphagia requiring dilation in the MSA group (9.3% vs 6.6% fundoplication). There were 13 reoperations in the MSA group and 12 in the LNF group. The cause of reoperation was device removal in 12 of the MSA patients. Importantly, the hospital length of stay ranged from 13 to 48 hours in the MSA group and from 26 to 48 hours in the fundoplication group.

MAGNETIC SPHINCTER AUGMENTATION VERSUS OPTIMAL MEDICAL THERAPY

In addition to comparing outcomes of MSA with fundoplication, it was important to compare MSA with optimal medical therapy directly. The CALIBER trial randomized 152 patients with persistent, moderate to severe reflux symptoms after daily PPI use to either MSA or twice-daily PPI, with the option of crossing over to the MSA group at 6 months.[33] At 6-month follow-up, 89% of MSA patients reported relief of their GERD-related symptoms versus 10% of PPI patients ($P<.001$). Ninety-one percent of the MSA patients were off PPIs (**Fig. 12**). Based on 24-hour pH impedance testing, there were significantly fewer reflux episodes with MSA than PPI (22.5 vs 49 respectively; $P<.001$). There were no statistically significant differences in DeMeester scores or mean esophageal acid exposure between the two groups.

SAFETY AND ADVERSE EVENTS

Most of the initial cohort studies examining MSA were small. Given the rare occurrence of adverse events with MSA, a true estimate of the incidence of safety issues was unknown. To further quantify the rate of adverse events, a review of the first 1000 MSA implants in 82 hospitals worldwide was conducted by Lipham and colleagues[34] in 2015. There were no intraoperative complications, and the 30-day readmission rate was 1.3%. There were reoperations in 3.4% and endoscopic dilatations in 5.6% of patients. These reoperations were mostly for persistent dysphagia. The rate of device erosion was 0.1% (**Table 3**).

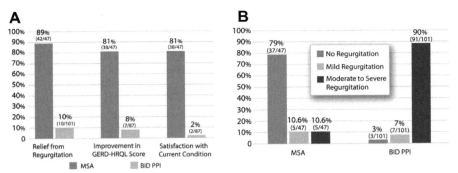

Fig. 12. (*A*) Percentage of patients with relief from regurgitation, improvement in GERD-HRQL score, or satisfaction with current condition, for MSA and twice-daily (BID) PPI groups. (*B*) Percentage of patients treated with MSA or twice-daily PPIs at the 6-month end point with no, mild, or moderate to severe regurgitation. (*From* Bell R, Lipham J, Louie B, Williams V, Luketich J, Hill M, et al. Laparoscopic magnetic sphincter augmentation versus double-dose proton pump inhibitors for management of moderate-to-severe regurgitation in GERD: a randomized controlled trial. Gastrointestinal Endoscopy. 2019;89(1):14-22; with permission.)

An additional safety study was conducted by Smith and colleagues[35] to include a larger cohort of 3282 patients. Researchers found a device removal prevalence of 2.7%. Dysphagia and persistence of reflux symptoms were the first and second most common reasons for removal, respectively. Fifty-seven percent of these removals occurred within the first year after surgery. There were no perforations or migrations. The prevalence of erosions was 0.15%.

In addition, one of the important safety concerns with MSA is the contraindication of its use with MRI. The original LINX device was compatible with MRIs up to 0.7 T. There were concerns of the device becoming demagnetized in a stronger magnetic field, leading to loss of its efficacy. However, the need for device removal for MRI was rare, even with use of the old device. A study published in 2014 analyzing the safety

Table 3
Device removals from Lipham and colleagues[34] (2015)

Reason for Device Removal	Removal ≤90 d After Implant		Removal ≥90 d After Implant	
	No. of Patients	% of Total Implants (n/1048)	No. of Patients	% of Total Implants (n/1048)
Dysphagia	16	1.5	7	0.7
GERD symptoms	0	0	7	0.7
Pain	1	0.1	2	0.2
Vomiting	0	0	1	0.1
MRI planned	0	0	1	0.1
Erosion	0	0	1	0.1
Overall	17	1.6	19	1.8

From Lipham JC, Taiganides PA, Louie BE, Ganz RA, Demeester TR. Safety analysis of first 1000 patients treated with magnetic sphincter augmentation for gastroesophageal reflux disease. Diseases of the Esophagus 2015;28 (4):305-11; with permission.

of the first 1000 devices implanted identified 19 device removals in total.[34] Only 1 of these was caused by need for MRI. The article by Smith and colleagues[35] mentioned earlier found only 0.09% of 3282 patients had a device removal because of need for MRI. In 2015, a new version of the device was approved for use in MRI machines up to 1.5 T.[23] The new magnetic beads have a higher resistance to being demagnetized. This development has largely resolved the issue of harm or demagnetization associated with the use of the LINX device, because 89% of all MRI machines in the United States do not have a strength greater than 1.5 T.[36]

EXPANDING THE INDICATIONS FOR MAGNETIC SPHINCTER AUGMENTATION

After establishing the comparative efficacy and safety of the device, the next broad direction for research in MSA was to consider whether the technology would be effective in patients with more severe forms of GERD. This group included patients with larger hiatal hernias, Barrett's esophagus, prior esophageal or gastric surgery (fundoplications), and so forth. These considerations are listed by the manufacturer as some of the general precautions surgeons should consider in choosing appropriate patients for MSA.

Patients with concurrent hiatal hernias larger than 3 cm were originally excluded from receiving an MSA. However, with an effective hiatal dissection and cruroplasty, it seemed reasonable that the device would still be effective and would not migrate into the chest. Therefore, several investigators decided to perform MSA with concurrent hiatal hernia repair.

A retrospective study by Rona and colleagues[37] included 192 patients, 57 of whom had concurrent hiatal hernias larger than 3 cm. Hiatal hernia repair followed by MSA was performed during the same operation in these patients. At a median follow-up time of 20 months, there was a significantly better postoperative GERD-HRQL score in the patients who had large hiatal hernias (3.6 vs 5.6, $P = .027$). This finding means that patients who required concomitant hiatal hernia repair felt better than their counterparts who did not require a concomitant hernia repair. There were no intraoperative or postoperative complications, and only 3 patients required device removal. The percentage of patients who required postoperative intervention for dysphagia (13.5% vs 17.9%, $P = .522$) and the incidence of symptom resolution or improvement (98.1% vs 91.3%, $P = .118$) did not reach statistical significance. This finding showed that MSA is as effective in patients with larger hiatal hernias.

The same cohort of patients with MSA and hiatal hernia repair were followed for a mean of 19 months (range, 1–39 months). In addition to symptom resolution, a main focus of this study was on the incidence of recurrent hiatal hernias. In terms of symptom resolution, 89% of patients remained off PPIs and 97% of patients reported clinical improvement. Only 2 hiatal hernia recurrences were identified postoperatively based on follow-up imaging. There were 6 patients with persistent dysphagia. Four of these patients resolved their dysphagia after a single endoscopic balloon dilatation. The remaining 2 had their devices removed.[38]

Buckley and colleagues[39] compared 200 separate patients who underwent concurrent hiatal hernia repair with MSA. All patients in this study had a hiatal hernia of at least 3 cm. The GERD-HRQL scores improved from an average of 26 preoperatively to 2 at a median follow-up of 258 days. Ninety-four percent of patients no longer required PPIs. There were 3 patients who had recurrence of their hiatal hernias at 1 year.

As mentioned earlier, another precaution for MSA is in patients with Barrett's esophagus. Recently published data suggest that there is regression of Barrett's esophagus following placement of a LINX device.[40] In a retrospective review of 443 patients undergoing MSA at a single institution, 86 patients were identified with Barrett's preoperatively. At a median of 1.2 years of follow-up, 71.6% of patients had no residual Barrett's identified on biopsies taken of the esophagus. Patients were more likely to have regression if their initial Barrett's segment was ultrashort (1 cm) or if their postoperative DeMeester score was less than 14.72.

Warren and colleagues[30] analyzed 170 patients in multivariate logistic regression to determine which factors were more likely associated with predicting an excellent or good outcome after MSA. Here the terms excellent and good refer to GERD-HRQL scores of less than 5 and 6 to 15 respectively. Patients with good outcomes were also allowed to have Los Angeles grade A esophagitis. Potential covariates entered into the model were BMI, structurally defective LES, Hill grade, hiatal hernia necessitating repair, and preoperative LES residual pressure. Of these, BMI greater than 35 (odds ratio [OR] = 0.05, 0.003–0.78; P = .03), structurally defective LES (OR = 0.37, 0.13–0.99; P = .05), and preoperative LES residual pressure (OR = 0.89, 0.80–0.98; P = .02) were statistically significant for chances of a poor outcome.

DEVICE REMOVALS

Although many studies have described removal rates of the device, the technique of device removal was not described, nor were in-depth analyses of device removals conducted, given their rarity. Asti and colleagues[41] were the first to describe their surgical technique for device removal. Tatum and colleagues[42] described indications and outcomes for 24 separate removals. Fifty-four percent were removed for refractory GERD symptoms, 33% of devices were removed for dysphagia, and 8% of the removals were for erosions. Interestingly, 42% of patients after removal had no additional antireflux surgery, even though they elected to have their device removed for persistent reflux symptoms.

CONTROVERSIES

One current controversy in MSA is how to properly size the esophagus and choose the appropriately sized device. The current protocol is to place a LINX device that is 2 sizes larger than the point at which the magnetic seal came apart on the sizing tool. A recently published study by Ayazi and colleagues[20] suggested that surgeons may be sizing the device too small. A study of 380 patients at a single center found that the size of the device was associated with whether the patient would eventually develop persistent dysphagia necessitating an endoscopic dilatation. However, device size did not reach statistical significance with regard to the overall rates of dysphagia. Nevertheless, researchers saw an absolute decrease in the amount of postoperative dysphagia when they began using a larger LINX device for each patient (**Fig. 13**). As a result, and in an attempt to minimize postoperative dysphagia, the current trend is for surgeons to place a LINX device that is 3 (vs 2) sizes larger than the point at which the magnetic seal comes apart.

ADDITIONAL NOVEL STUDIES

Transient postoperative dysphagia is very common after MSA, seen in two-thirds of patients in some of the early trials. Prolonged postoperative dysphagia is a common reason for device removal. The aforementioned study by Ayazi and colleagues[20] also examined other risk factors for dysphagia. At 11.5 months, 15% of patients experienced persistent dysphagia. Thirty-one percent of these patients required balloon dilatation and 40% of these patients had resolution of their symptoms after 1 dilatation. Interestingly, patients who had persistent dysphagia did not differ from other MSA patients based on their LES resting and residual pressures. In a multivariate

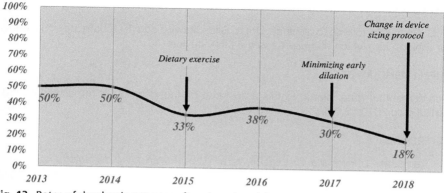

Fig. 13. Rates of dysphagia per year after changing sizing protocol. (*From* Ayazi S, Zheng P, Zaidi AH, Chovanec K, Chowdhury N, Salvitti M, et al. Magnetic Sphincter Augmentation and Postoperative Dysphagia: Characterization, Clinical Risk Factors, and Management. Journal of Gastrointestinal Surgery. 2019; with permission.)

logistic regression model, preoperative dysphagia, peristalsis in less than 80% of swallows, and the absence of a large paraesophageal hernia were significantly associated with postoperative dysphagia. The investigators commented that endoscopic intervention within the first 8 weeks after surgery does not seem to alleviate any dysphagia and may worsen the symptoms.

A noteworthy study was published in 2018 by Tatum and colleagues[43] comparing the degree of hiatal dissection done in concurrence with MSA placement. Patients who had a more thorough dissection of the phrenoesophageal ligament in order to repair a large hiatal hernia defect were compared with patients who did not require this dissection because they did not have a large hiatal hernia. Patients had a higher rate of delayed-onset dysphagia, and a higher rate of hiatal hernia recurrence in the minimal dissection group, which was statistically significant. The researchers hypothesized that the diaphragm contributes significantly to the antireflux mechanism, which is why those patients who received concurrent repair of their larger hiatal hernias did better than those with smaller hernias without repair.

In addition, there were initially concerns with the overall cost of MSA versus traditional fundoplication. In a retrospective review of 119 patients, the total charges for MSA, including hospitalization, were $48,491. The cost of hospitalization for LNF was $50,111. These differences were not statistically significant ($P = .506$).[44] Researchers discovered that the increased cost of the device was offset by the cost for medications, laboratory tests, radiology, and longer hospital stay associated with LF.

SUMMARY

MSA with the LINX device has revitalized antireflux surgery, providing excellent outcomes for many patients. The device allows a technically easier and standardized operation with fewer side effects, equal efficacy, and similar costs. New research is focusing on MSA in patients who have reflux following sleeve gastrectomy, comparison of MSA with endoluminal antireflux procedures, and methods to improve the reflux barrier by strengthening diaphragmatic repairs. Regardless of what this new research shows, LINX is now established as an excellent option for foregut surgeons to treat GERD.

DISCLOSURE

Dr C. Dunn has nothing to disclose. Drs N. Bildzukewicz and J. Lipham are consultants for Ethicon Inc, which manufactures the LINX device.

SUPPLEMENTARY DATA

Supplementary data related to this article can be found online at https://doi.org/10.1016/j.giec.2019.12.010.

REFERENCES

1. Yamasaki T, Hemond C, Eisa M, et al. The changing epidemiology of gastro-esophageal reflux disease: are patients getting younger? J Neurogastroenterol Motil 2018;24(4):559–69.
2. Rubenstein JH, Chen JW. Epidemiology of gastroesophageal reflux disease. Gastroenterol Clin North Am 2014;43(1):1–14.
3. El-Serag H, Becher A, Jones R. Systematic review: persistent reflux symptoms on proton pump inhibitor therapy in primary care and community studies. Aliment Pharmacol Ther 2010;32(6):720–37.
4. Fass R, Shapiro M, Dekel R, et al. Systematic review: proton-pump inhibitor failure in gastro-oesophageal reflux disease - where next? Aliment Pharmacol Ther 2005;22(2):79–94.
5. Ganz RA, Edmundowicz SA, Taiganides PA, et al. Long-term outcomes of patients receiving a magnetic sphincter augmentation device for gastroesophageal reflux. Clin Gastroenterol Hepatol 2016;14(5):671–7.
6. Kessing BF, Broeders JAJL, Vinke N, et al. Gas-related symptoms after antireflux surgery. Surg Endosc 2013;27(10):3739–47.
7. Castelijns PSS, Ponten JEH, Vd Poll MCG, et al. Quality of life after Nissen fundoplication in patients with gastroesophageal reflux disease: comparison between long- and short-term follow-up. J Minim Access Surg 2018;14(3):213–20.
8. Finks JF, Wei Y, Birkmeyer JD. The rise and fall of antireflux surgery in the United States. Surg Endosc 2006;20(11):1698–701.
9. Hershcovici T, Fass R. Step-by-step management of refractory gastresophageal reflux disease. Dis Esophagus 2013;26(1):27–36.
10. Vakil N, Shaw M, Kirby R. Clinical effectiveness of laparoscopic fundoplication in a U.S. community. Am J Med 2003;114(1):1–5.
11. Ganz RA. A modern magnetic implant for gastroesophageal reflux disease. Clin Gastroenterol Hepatol 2017;15(9):1326–37.
12. Al-Mansour MR, Perry KA, Hazey JW. The current status of magnetic sphincter augmentation in the management of gastroesophageal reflux disease. Ann Laparosc Endosc Surg 2017;2(9).
13. Vakil N, van Zanten SV, Kahrilas P, et al. The Montreal definition and classification of gastroesophageal reflux disease: a global evidence-based consensus. Am J Gastroenterol 2006;101(8):1900–20.
14. Numans ME, Lau J, De Wit NJ, et al. Short-term treatment with proton-pump inhibitors as a test for gastroesophageal reflux disease. Ann Intern Med 2004;140(7):518.
15. Hunt R, Armstrong D, Katelaris P, et al. World Gastroenterology Organisation global guidelines: GERD global perspective on gastroesophageal reflux disease. J Clin Gastroenterol 2017;51(6):467–78.

16. Lundell LR, Dent J, Bennett JR, et al. Endoscopic assessment of oesophagitis: clinical and functional correlates and further validation of the Los Angeles classification. Gut 1999;45(2):172–80.
17. Hill LD, Kozarek RA, Kraemer SJM, et al. The gastroesophageal flap valve: in vitro and in vivo observations. Gastrointest Endosc 1996;44(5):541–7.
18. Schwameis K, Lin B, Roman J, et al. Is pH testing necessary before antireflux surgery in patients with endoscopic erosive esophagitis? J Gastrointest Surg 2018; 22(1):8–12.
19. Alicuben ET, Bildzukewicz N, Samakar K, et al. Routine esophageal manometry is not useful in patients with normal videoesophagram. Surg Endosc 2019;33(5): 1650–3.
20. Ayazi S, Zheng P, Zaidi AH, et al. Magnetic sphincter augmentation and postoperative dysphagia: characterization, clinical risk factors, and management. J Gastrointest Surg 2019. https://doi.org/10.1007/s11605-019-04331-9.
21. Bonavina L, Saino GI, Bona D, et al. Magnetic augmentation of the lower esophageal sphincter: results of a feasibility clinical trial. J Gastrointest Surg 2008; 12(12):2133–40.
22. Bonavina L, DeMeester T, Fockens P, et al. Laparoscopic sphincter augmentation device eliminates reflux symptoms and normalizes esophageal acid exposure: one- and 2-year results of a feasibility trial. Ann Surg 2010;252(5):857–62.
23. Asti E, Aiolfi A, Lazzari V, et al. Magnetic sphincter augmentation for gastroesophageal reflux disease: review of clinical studies. Updates Surg 2018;70(3):323–30.
24. Ganz RA, Peters JH, Horgan S, et al. Esophageal sphincter device for gastroesophageal reflux disease. N Engl J Med 2013;368(8):719–27.
25. Bonavina L, Saino G, Bona D, et al. One hundred consecutive patients treated with magnetic sphincter augmentation for gastroesophageal reflux disease: 6 years of clinical experience from a single center. J Am Coll Surg 2013;217(4): 577–85.
26. Reynolds JL, Zehetner J, Wu P, et al. Laparoscopic magnetic sphincter augmentation vs laparoscopic nissen fundoplication: a matched-pair analysis of 100 patients. J Am Coll Surg 2015;221(1):123–8.
27. Riegler M, Schoppman SF, Bonavina L, et al. Magnetic sphincter augmentation and fundoplication for GERD in clinical practice: one-year results of a multicenter, prospective observational study. Surg Endosc 2015;29(5):1123–9.
28. Sheu EG, Nau P, Nath B, et al. A comparative trial of laparoscopic magnetic sphincter augmentation and Nissen fundoplication. Surg Endosc 2015;29(3): 505–9.
29. Louie BE, Farivar AS, Shultz D, et al. Short-term outcomes using magnetic sphincter augmentation versus nissen fundoplication for medically resistant gastroesophageal reflux disease. Ann Thorac Surg 2014;98(2):498–505.
30. Warren HF, Reynolds JL, Lipham JC, et al. Multi-institutional outcomes using magnetic sphincter augmentation versus Nissen fundoplication for chronic gastroesophageal reflux disease. Surg Endosc 2016;30(8):3289–96.
31. Asti E, Bonitta G, Lovece A, et al. Longitudinal comparison of quality of life in patients undergoing laparoscopic Toupet fundoplication versus magnetic sphincter augmentation: observational cohort study with propensity score analysis. Medicine (Baltimore) 2016;95(30):e4366.
32. Aiolfi A, Asti E, Bernardi D, et al. Early results of magnetic sphincter augmentation versus fundoplication for gastroesophageal reflux disease: systematic review and meta-analysis. Int J Surg 2018;52:82–8.

33. Bell R, Lipham J, Louie B, et al. Laparoscopic magnetic sphincter augmentation versus double-dose proton pump inhibitors for management of moderate-to-severe regurgitation in GERD: a randomized controlled trial. Gastrointest Endosc 2019;89(1):14–22.

34. Lipham JC, Taiganides PA, Louie BE, et al. Safety analysis of first 1000 patients treated with magnetic sphincter augmentation for gastroesophageal reflux disease. Dis Esophagus 2015;28(4):305–11.

35. Smith CD, Ganz RA, Lipham JC, et al. Lower esophageal sphincter augmentation for gastroesophageal reflux disease: the safety of a modern implant. J Laparoendosc Adv Surg Tech A 2017. https://doi.org/10.1089/lap.2017.0025.

36. Diagnostic Imaging with LINX. Secondary Diagnostic Imaging with LINX. Available at: https://www.linxforlife.com/mri-info. Accessed September 8, 2019.

37. Rona KA, Reynolds J, Schwameis K, et al. Efficacy of magnetic sphincter augmentation in patients with large hiatal hernias. Surg Endosc 2017;31(5): 2096–102.

38. Rona KA, Tatum JM, Zehetner J, et al. Hiatal hernia recurrence following magnetic sphincter augmentation and posterior cruroplasty: intermediate-term outcomes. Surg Endosc 2018;32(7):3374–9.

39. Buckley FP, Bell RCW, Freeman K, et al. Favorable results from a prospective evaluation of 200 patients with large hiatal hernias undergoing LINX magnetic sphincter augmentation. Surg Endosc 2018;32(4):1762–8.

40. Alicuben ET, Tatum JM, Bildzukewicz N, et al. Regression of intestinal metaplasia following magnetic sphincter augmentation device placement. Surg Endosc 2019;33(2):576–9.

41. Asti E, Siboni S, Lazzari V, et al. Removal of the magnetic sphincter augmentation device: surgical technique and results of a single-center cohort study. Ann Surg 2017;265(5):941–5.

42. Tatum JM, Alicuben E, Bildzukewicz N, et al. Removing the magnetic sphincter augmentation device: operative management and outcomes. Surg Endosc 2019;33(8):2663–9.

43. Tatum JM, Alicuben E, Bildzukewicz N, et al. Minimal versus obligatory dissection of the diaphragmatic hiatus during magnetic sphincter augmentation surgery. Surg Endosc 2019;33(3):782–8.

44. Reynolds JL, Zehetner J, Nieh A, et al. Charges, outcomes, and complications: a comparison of magnetic sphincter augmentation versus laparoscopic Nissen fundoplication for the treatment of GERD. Surg Endosc 2016;30(8):3225–30.

Refractory Gastroesophageal Reflux Disease and Functional Heartburn

Stuart Jon Spechler, MD

KEYWORDS

- Gastroesophageal reflux disease • Reflux hypersensitivity • Functional heartburn
- Fundoplication • Proton pump inhibitor • Magnetic sphincter augmentation

KEY POINTS

- Heartburn can be considered PPI refractory when it does not respond to double-dose PPI therapy (first dose taken 30–60 minutes before breakfast, second dose taken 30–60 minutes before dinner).
- PPIs can eliminate all endoscopic and histologic evidence of eosinophilic esophagitis, and therefore PPIs should be stopped for 3 to 4 weeks if possible before performing diagnostic endoscopy for patients with PPI-refractory heartburn.
- Reflux hypersensitivity is diagnosed when systematic workup reveals no esophageal endoscopic, histologic, or motility abnormalities to account for heartburn, and esophageal MII-pH monitoring reveals normal esophageal acid exposure with a positive symptom index (SI) or positive symptom association probability (SAP) for heartburn.
- Functional heartburn is diagnosed when systematic workup reveals no esophageal endoscopic, histologic, or motility abnormalities to account for heartburn, and esophageal MII-pH monitoring reveals normal esophageal acid exposure with a negative SI or negative SAP for heartburn.

PROBLEMS WITH DEFINING "REFRACTORY GASTROESOPHAGEAL REFLUX DISEASE"

There is no clear consensus regarding the precise definition of the term refractory GERD. GERD can be complicated by reflux esophagitis and peptic esophageal strictures, which occasionally can be difficult to treat and hence might be considered refractory. Patients with GERD typically complain of heartburn and regurgitation, symptoms that usually respond well to treatment but sometimes do not, and GERD can have many notoriously difficult-to-treat atypical symptoms, such as chest pain, chronic cough, hoarseness, and throat clearing.[1] Furthermore, there are many

Division of Gastroenterology, Center for Esophageal Diseases, Baylor University Medical Center at Dallas, The Center for Esophageal Research, Baylor Scott & White Research Institute, 3500 Gaston Avenue, 2 Hoblitzelle, Suite 250, Dallas, TX 75246, USA
E-mail address: sjspechler@aol.com

Gastrointest Endoscopy Clin N Am 30 (2020) 343–359
https://doi.org/10.1016/j.giec.2019.12.003
1052-5157/20/© 2019 Elsevier Inc. All rights reserved.

different types of treatments for GERD, including lifestyle modifications, antacids, alginates, acid-reducing medications, such as proton pump inhibitors (PPIs) and histamine H_2 receptor antagonists (H_2RAs), antireflux medications, such as baclofen, endoscopic procedures, such as transoral incisionless fundoplication (TIF), and surgical procedures, such as fundoplication. Although the term refractory GERD conceivably could be applied to any one or combination of the above problems that do not respond to any number of procedures or medications given for different durations in variable dosages, the term usually is used for symptoms that are assumed to be due to GERD and that have not responded to a trial of PPI therapy.

The PPIs are the most effective available medical treatment for GERD, and the US Food and Drug Administration (FDA) approves once-daily PPI dosing for patients with GERD. The FDA does not approve double-dose PPI therapy and, for patients whose symptoms are refractory to the conventional PPI dosage, doubling the dose usually achieves only modest additional therapeutic benefit.[2] Nevertheless, patients with GERD generally are not considered "PPI-refractory" until they have been on a double dose of PPIs with the first dose taken 30 to 60 minutes before breakfast and the second dose taken 30 to 60 minutes before dinner. Sifrim and Zerbib have proposed that patients with troublesome heartburn and regurgitation who do not respond to 12 weeks of double-dose PPIs can be considered to have PPI-refractory reflux symptoms.[3] Alternatively, Yadlapati and Delay have defined "PPI-refractory GERD" as persistent troublesome GERD symptoms with objective evidence of GERD after 8 weeks of double-dose PPI therapy.[4] These definitions, which might be useful as criteria for clinical studies, might be too restrictive for rigorous application in clinical practice.

PPIs can heal reflux esophagitis in the large majority of cases,[5] but they are considerably less effective for eliminating GERD symptoms, which allegedly persist in up to 40% of patients who take PPIs for GERD.[3] Indeed, PPI-refractory GERD is the most common reason for GERD-related referrals to gastroenterologists.[6] However, a careful medical history often will reveal that what patients perceive as persistent "GERD symptoms" during PPI treatment either are not GERD symptoms at all (eg, bloating, early satiation) or are symptoms that can have multiple causes other than GERD (eg, cough, hoarseness, throat clearing), and hence might not be due to GERD. Although heartburn and regurgitation, the cardinal symptoms of GERD, are far more likely to respond to PPIs than the atypical symptoms, a PPI response is neither a sensitive nor specific test for GERD.[7] In 1 study in which 299 primary care patients with heartburn, regurgitation, or chest pain were treated empirically with esomeprazole 40 mg every day for 2 weeks, only 67% of those with objective evidence of GERD (by endoscopy or esophageal pH monitoring) experienced a symptomatic response to this "PPI test," whereas 60% of those with no objective evidence of GERD nevertheless had a positive PPI test (ie, a symptomatic response to PPIs).[8]

Among the atypical GERD symptoms, noncardiac chest pain seems to have the best response to PPIs, especially for patients who also have objective evidence of abnormal acid reflux.[1] A systematic review of randomized controlled trials of PPIs for chest pain found that they were beneficial in 56% to 85% of patients with chest pain who had objective evidence of GERD by pH monitoring or endoscopy, but in only 0% to 17% of patients without such objective evidence.[9] The efficacy of PPIs for atypical, extraesophageal GERD symptoms, such as throat clearing, hoarseness, and chronic cough is much less clear and much more controversial. Some observational studies have documented PPI efficacy in relieving these symptoms, but controlled trials have not consistently demonstrated a benefit of PPIs over placebo for patients with such "extraesophageal GERD."[10–14] Furthermore, although physicians often assume (often with little or no evidence) that GERD is the cause of these extraesophageal symptoms, that assumption is incorrect in many, if not most cases.[15]

Laryngopharyngeal reflux (LPR) disease is an especially contentious condition for which there is no diagnostic "gold standard," and no reliably effective treatment.[16] Even the laryngoscopic demonstration of LPR is weak evidence that GERD is the underlying condition. In 1 study of 52 healthy volunteers (with no history of GERD or ear, nose, and throat problems) who had flexible videolaryngologic examinations reviewed by experts, at least 1 sign of LPR was detected in 93% of those healthy study subjects.[17] Thus, when managing patients with atypical, extraesophageal symptoms, clinicians should be cautious about making a diagnosis of refractory LPR disease, especially if there is only weak evidence that GERD is the underlying cause. Use of the terms refractory GERD or "refractory LPR" in such cases can bias clinical decision making, because the underlying assumption for the use of both terms is that GERD is the cause of the problems, and this can result in inappropriate use of invasive GERD treatments for patients whose symptoms are not due to GERD. A detailed discussion of the diagnosis and management of LPR disease is beyond the scope of this article and is covered extensively in Caroline M. Barrett and colleagues' article, "Laryngopharyngeal Reflux and Atypical Gastroesophageal Reflux Disease," in this issue. The reader is also referred to an excellent recent review of this topic.[16] The remainder of this report will deal with the management of patients who have the typical GERD symptoms of heartburn and regurgitation that are refractory to PPI therapy.

PROTON PUMP INHIBITOR PHARMACODYNAMICS AND PREPARATIONS

Because PPIs are vulnerable to degradation by gastric acid, most are manufactured with an acid-resistant enteric coating that delays their release and absorption. Also, all of the PPIs are prodrugs that must be converted into an active, sulfenamide form by the acid produced by the proton pumps (H^+, K^+-ATPases) of gastric parietal cells. This sulfenamide form disables those proton pumps by binding to them covalently. Because PPIs can bind only to proton pumps that are actively secreting acid, PPIs should be dosed before meals to provide maximal acid suppression. In the fasting state, fewer than 10% of gastric proton pumps are active, whereas approximately 70% are active when stimulated by meals.[18] Thus, PPIs should be taken 30 to 60 minutes before meals, the optimal time to enable their absorption and transport to actively secreting parietal cells. One study of 100 patients with persistent GERD symptoms on PPI therapy found that 54 took the medication incorrectly (21 >60 minutes before meals, 16 after meals, 15 at bedtime, 2 as needed).[19] Thus, it is important to ask patients with PPI-refractory GERD how they are taking their PPIs, and to stress the importance of taking them 30 to 60 minutes before meals. A recent study reported in abstract form found that approximately 11.5% of patients referred to Veterans Affairs GI clinics for PPI-refractory heartburn responded to this simple clinical maneuver.[20,21]

Although all available PPIs are effective for healing reflux esophagitis when given in their standard dosages, the acid suppression potency of the different PPI preparations varies widely. If relative acid suppression potencies of individual PPIs (based on their effects on mean 24-hour intragastric pH) are standardized to omeprazole in terms of "omeprazole equivalents" ([OEs], with omeprazole having an OE of 1.00), the relative potencies of standard-dose pantoprazole, lansoprazole, omeprazole, esomeprazole, and rabeprazole have been estimated at 0.23, 0.90, 1.00, 1.60, and 1.82 OEs, respectively.[22,23] Thus, 4 pantoprazole tablets are needed to achieve the acid-suppressing capability of 1 omeprazole tablet. Individual patients also can exhibit considerable variability in their response to different PPIs.[24] These data suggest that it might be useful to switch patients with PPI-refractory symptoms from one PPI to another, preferably more potent one, although there are few clinical data that support the clinical efficacy of this maneuver.

PROTON PUMP INHIBITOR-REFRACTORY HEARTBURN

Heartburn, the most typical and most frequent symptom of GERD, can be defined as a burning sensation in the retrosternal area.[25] Patients frequently relate that the burning sensation moves up the chest and that it is relieved by antacids. When describing heartburn, patients typically wave an open hand over the sternum, unlike patients with angina pectoris who might hold a clenched fist over the left chest when describing their pain (Levine sign). The physician's first step in the evaluation of a patient with PPI-refractory heartburn is to ask the patient for a detailed description of the symptom. A patient's concept of what the term "heartburn" means can differ dramatically from the physician's concept and, when asked for a description, many patients who say or were told that they have heartburn will describe a symptom that cannot originate from the esophagus.[26] However, even if the description is consistent with the heartburn of GERD, heartburn is by no means specific for GERD. Patients with eosinophilic esophagitis (EoE) or esophageal motility disorders, such as achalasia can experience heartburn, and balloon distention of the esophagus can elicit retrosternal burning typical of heartburn.[27]

Five major mechanisms might explain heartburn that does not respond to PPIs[28]: (1) the PPIs have not normalized esophageal acid exposure; (2) the PPIs have normalized esophageal acid exposure but there is reflux hypersensitivity, the condition in which persistent "physiologic" reflux events (acidic or nonacidic) evoke heartburn[29]; (3) the sensation of heartburn is caused by an esophageal disorder other than GERD, such as EoE or achalasia; (4) the sensation of heartburn is caused by an extraesophageal disorder, such as heart or gallbladder disease; or (5) there is functional heartburn, meaning that the sensation of heartburn is not caused by GERD, reflux events, or any other identifiable histopathologic, motility, or structural abnormality.[29] A rigorous, systematic evaluation that includes careful medical history, endoscopy with esophageal biopsy, esophageal manometry, and esophageal multichannel intraluminal impedance (MII)-pH monitoring can distinguish among these mechanisms as discussed below.

Proton Pump Inhibitors Have Not Normalized Esophageal Acid Exposure

Patients who have a severe reflux diathesis, such as those with long-segment Barrett's esophagus, often have persistently abnormal acid reflux despite high-dose PPI therapy. In 1 study of 31 patients with long-segment Barrett's esophagus treated with esomeprazole 40 mg twice a day, 24-hour esophageal pH monitoring demonstrated persistently abnormal acid reflux in 23%.[30] However, PPI-refractory heartburn is unusual in Barrett's patients, even when abnormal acid reflux persists during PPI therapy.[31] In other words, PPIs usually eliminate heartburn in patients with Barrett's esophagus even when they do not normalize esophageal acid exposure.

Approximately one-third of patients with PPI-refractory GERD symptoms who are treated with PPIs in standard, once-daily dosage will have persistently abnormal acid reflux exposure found on esophageal pH monitoring studies.[32,33] However, abnormal acid reflux is decidedly unusual in patients who take PPIs twice-daily. In 1 study of patients with PPI-refractory GERD symptoms on twice-daily PPIs, abnormal esophageal acid exposure was found in only 7% of 52 patients with typical GERD symptoms, and in only 1% of patients with extraesophageal GERD symptoms.[32] Thus, persistently abnormal acid reflux is an uncommon cause of PPI-refractory heartburn.

Proton Pump Inhibitors Have Normalized Esophageal Acid Exposure, but There Is Reflux Hypersensitivity

By convention, esophageal pH monitoring identifies acid reflux when esophageal pH values fall below 4. In contrast, esophageal impedance monitoring detects the reflux of all gastric material whether it is acidic (pH <4), weakly acidic (pH >4 to <7), or alkaline (pH >7). In the era before esophageal impedance monitoring was available, the term "acid hypersensitivity" was used to describe patients who had normal esophageal acid exposure by esophageal pH monitoring, but in whom "physiologic" episodes of acid reflux were associated with heartburn. More recent esophageal MII-pH monitoring studies have established that reflux episodes with pH >4 also can be associated with heartburn. Consequently, the term acid hypersensitivity has been replaced by the term "reflux hypersensitivity," the condition in which patients with normal esophageal acid exposure have reflux episodes (acidic, weakly acidic, or alkaline) associated with heartburn.[29] It has been estimated that 28% to 36% of patients who do not respond to twice-daily PPI therapy have reflux hypersensitivity.[1]

The mechanisms through which reflux episodes cause heartburn are poorly understood. It has been proposed that refluxed acid (pH <4) causes heartburn by activating acid-sensitive nociceptors in the esophageal epithelium.[31] The mechanism whereby the reflux of less acidic material causes heartburn is even less clear. Perhaps weakly acidic refluxate (pH >4 and <7) can trigger the same nociceptors activated by more strongly acidic material. Alternatively, the reflux of irritants other than acid (eg, bile salts) might trigger the nociceptors that convey heartburn, or large-volume reflux might cause esophageal distention that activates those nociceptors. It also has been proposed that reflux can result in sustained contractions of esophageal longitudinal muscle that elicit the sensations of heartburn and chest pain.[34,35]

The diagnosis of reflux hypersensitivity requires the demonstration of an association between reflux episodes and symptom episodes in patients who have normal esophageal acid exposure.[29] Esophageal pH or MII-pH monitoring studies typically use 2 indices to identify a significant association between reflux and symptom episodes: the symptom index (SI) and the symptom association probability (SAP). To calculate the SI, the total number of reflux episodes that are associated with symptom episodes is divided by the total number of symptom episodes recorded during the monitoring period.[36] If ≥50% of all symptom episodes are associated with an episode of reflux, then the SI is considered positive. The validity of the SI has been questioned for several reasons, but primarily because it does not consider the total number of reflux events. For example, if a patient has 100 episodes of acid reflux during the monitoring period but only 1 symptom episode, and that symptom episode by chance happens to correspond with one of the 100 acid reflux episodes, then that patient would have an SI of 100%, spuriously suggesting a very strong association between symptoms and reflux episodes.

The SAP was developed in an attempt to circumvent the shortcomings of the SI.[37] To determine the SAP, the 24-hour monitoring period is divided into 720 two-minute increments, and each increment is evaluated for the occurrence of reflux and symptom episodes. Then, a Fisher exact test is performed to determine a P value for the probability that the reflux and symptom events are randomly distributed. The SAP is determined by subtracting the calculated P value from 1, and the remainder is multiplied by 100%. A positive SAP is defined as greater than 95%, meaning that the chance that reflux and symptom events are randomly distributed throughout the monitoring period has a *P* value of less than 0.05. In other words, a positive SAP identifies a significant association between reflux and symptom episodes. Unfortunately for clinical purposes, SAP and SI results do not always agree and, despite the theoretic advantages of the SAP, its clinical superiority over the SI has not been established unequivocally. In addition, the validity of the SAP for distinguishing reflux hypersensitivity from functional heartburn has been questioned.[38,39]

Heartburn Is Caused by an Esophageal Disorder Other than Gastroesophageal Reflux Disease

Esophageal inflammation of any cause conceivably might induce the retrosternal burning discomfort of heartburn, but EoE is the inflammatory disorder most likely to be confused with GERD. Patients with EoE commonly have a history of atopy, are younger than the typical patient with GERD, and usually present because of dysphagia and food impaction rather than heartburn. Nevertheless, confusion with GERD can arise, especially for patients whose major complaint is heartburn.[40] The characteristic endoscopic findings of EoE are esophageal exudates, rings, edema, furrows, and strictures, and the diagnosis is established when esophageal biopsies show greater than 15 eosinophils per high power field and other causes of esophageal eosinophilia are excluded. The esophagus can appear endoscopically normal in approximately 10% of patients with EoE, so esophageal biopsies should be taken routinely in any patient having endoscopy for PPI-responsive heartburn irrespective of the endoscopic appearance of the esophagus.

Until recently, PPIs were used as a test to distinguish GERD from EoE with the assumption that only the acid-peptic disease (GERD) could respond to PPI therapy.[41] For patients with PPI-refractory heartburn, therefore, it was not common practice to stop PPIs before diagnostic endoscopy to look for EoE since PPI responsiveness was thought to exclude that diagnosis. More recent data have shown that EoE can respond to PPIs, and PPIs are now considered a treatment for EoE, not a diagnostic test for the condition.[42] Because it is now well established that PPIs can eliminate the endoscopic and histologic signs of EoE, it follows that an endoscopy performed for a patient on PPIs cannot rule out EoE. When EoE is a diagnostic consideration, as it is for patients with PPI-refractory heartburn, then PPIs should be discontinued for 3 to 4 weeks before diagnostic endoscopy whenever possible.[43] Stopping PPIs will also be helpful for determining the severity of GERD, since PPIs can also eliminate the endoscopic signs of reflux esophagitis. Indeed, it is not appropriate to make a diagnosis of nonerosive reflux disease (NERD) based on an endoscopy performed for patients taking PPIs. Patients with achalasia, an esophageal motility disorder that typically causes dysphagia, frequently complain of heartburn that can be confused with GERD.[44] In achalasia, loss of neurons in the wall of the esophagus results in inadequate lower esophageal sphincter (LES) relaxation with swallowing, and abnormal function in muscles of the esophageal body. It is not clear whether the sensation of heartburn in achalasia is caused by the abnormal esophageal motor activity, or by acid that might reflux into the esophagus when the LES finally does relax. Abnormal esophageal acid exposure has been documented in patients with achalasia, although it is not clear whether the acid in the esophagus is hydrochloric acid refluxed from the stomach, or lactic acid produced by the fermentation of carbohydrate retained in the achalasic esophagus.[45] Patients with achalasia can have PPI-refractory heartburn, a feature that occasionally has resulted in achalasia patients having Nissen fundoplications to treat heartburn mistakenly attributed to GERD. Nissen fundoplication can cause debilitating dysphagia in this setting.[46] Therefore, for patients considering fundoplication for the treatment of GERD, preoperative esophageal manometry is recommended to avoid this potentially devastating mistake.

Heartburn Is Caused by an Extraesophageal Disorder

Because both GERD and coronary artery diseases (CADs) are associated with obesity,[47] it is not surprising that obese patients with CAD frequently have GERD.[48] Angina can be described as burning in character and it is certainly conceivable that angina might be incorrectly diagnosed as heartburn due to GERD.[49] However, there is surprisingly little published documentation of this error. Patients can misunderstand what is meant by the term heartburn, and might mistakenly use that term for what are in fact typical anginal symptoms.[26] If such patients tell their physicians that they have heartburn, and the physicians take that history at face value without asking for a description of the heartburn, then angina due to CAD might well be confused with GERD. It is not clear how often angina causes retrosternal burning discomfort that could not be distinguished from the heartburn of GERD by a careful history. Nevertheless, since the consequences of misdiagnosing CAD as GERD can be catastrophic, clinicians should consider the possibility that CAD might cause a heartburn sensation that does not respond to PPIs, especially in older patients with other risk factors for CAD.

The pain of pancreatic or biliary tract disease does not respond to PPIs, and conceivably could be confused with heartburn if it is burning in character and referred to the epigastrium or lower chest. As is the case for angina due to CAD, however, it is not clear how often pancreaticobiliary disease causes retrosternal burning discomfort that a careful history could not distinguish from the heartburn of GERD. Nevertheless, clinicians should consider the possibility that pancreaticobiliary diseases might underlie PPI-refractory pain, especially in patients with other risk factors for those diseases.

FUNCTIONAL HEARTBURN

When the above mechanisms have been excluded, PPI-refractory heartburn can be considered functional.[29] Unfortunately, "functional" is a nonspecific and potentially stigmatizing term that has engendered considerable confusion and contention among experts over the years. In 1992, a group of such experts met in Rome to formulate a classification system for functional gastrointestinal disorders, and so devised the "Rome criteria" to codify gastrointestinal syndromes that were not from any named histopathologic, motility, or structural abnormality. Since then, there have been 3 more iterations of the Rome criteria, all struggling with use of the term functional. It has become clear that some patients with so-called functional disorders can have subtle histopathologic and physiologic abnormalities that have no specific names. Rome IV, the most recent iteration of the Rome criteria, discourages use of the term functional, and suggest that the traditional functional gastrointestinal disorders should instead be called "disorders of gut-brain interaction."[50] Nevertheless, Rome IV retains the term "functional heartburn" and, adding to the confusion, also deems reflux hypersensitivity to be a "functional gastrointestinal disorder."[29]

Rome IV defines functional heartburn as retrosternal burning discomfort or pain that is, refractory to "optimal antisecretory therapy" in the absence of GERD, histopathologic mucosal abnormalities, major motor disorders, or structural explanations.[29] Functional heartburn is distinguished from reflux hypersensitivity by esophageal pH or MII-pH monitoring studies that show no association between reflux episodes and heartburn episodes (ie, SI <50% and/or SAP ≤95%). It has been estimated that 29% to 39% of patients who do not respond to twice-daily PPI therapy have functional heartburn.[1] The mechanisms underlying functional heartburn are not known, but they seem to be unrelated to gastroesophageal reflux. Consequently, medications and procedures aimed at controlling reflux should not be prescribed for patients with functional heartburn, and treatment can focus on the use of neuromodulators or cognitive behavior therapy (see later discussion). Although Rome IV considers reflux hypersensitivity to be a functional disorder, a recent randomized trial of medical and surgical therapy for patients with PPI-refractory heartburn (so far reported only in abstract form) found that fundoplication was superior to medical treatment for highly selected patients with reflux hypersensitivity.[20]

REGURGITATION

PPIs inhibit gastric acid secretion but do nothing to correct the reflux diathesis underlying GERD.[51] Consequently, it is not surprising that PPIs have limited efficacy in relieving the typical GERD symptom of regurgitation. Experts at the Montreal consensus conference on GERD in 2006 defined regurgitation as "the perception of flow of refluxed gastric content into the mouth or hypopharynx."[25] However, the Reflux Disease Questionnaire (RDQ), a validated instrument used in the evaluation of patients with GERD, has describes 2 symptoms that can be considered regurgitation (1) an acid taste in the mouth and (2) unpleasant movement of material upward from the stomach. Studies that have used the RDQ found that regurgitation is a troublesome symptom in approximately 50% of patients with GERD, and that PPIs relieve regurgitation only marginally better than placebo.[14,52] For patients with PPI-refractory regurgitation as a predominant symptom, further medical therapy is notoriously ineffective and antireflux procedures are far better at relieving the symptom (see later discussion).

TREATMENTS OTHER THAN PROTON PUMP INHIBITORSS FOR PROTON PUMP INHIBITOR-REFRACTORY HEARTBURN THAT IS REFLUX RELATED
Antireflux Lifestyle Modifications

Antireflux lifestyle modifications (elevation of the head of the bed on 4″ to 6″ blocks, weight loss for overweight patients, avoiding recumbency for several hours after meals, avoiding bedtime snacks, and avoiding fatty foods, smoking and alcoholic beverages) were once considered first-line therapy for GERD, but their usefulness has dwindled since the introduction of PPIs into clinical practice in 1989. Only very limited data support the efficacy of these lifestyle modifications in controlling GERD symptoms at all, and data on their efficacy in patients with PPI-refractory GERD are virtually nonexistent. Nevertheless, it seems reasonable to try these modifications for patients with PPI-refractory GERD, especially those with reflux hypersensitivity or troublesome regurgitation who might benefit from modifications that reduce reflux episodes.

Baclofen

Transient LES relaxation (TLESR) is a major mechanism underlying episodes of gastroesophageal reflux in patients with GERD as well as in normal individuals.[53] Unlike the brief, appropriate LES relaxations induced by swallowing, TLESRs are not preceded by swallowing and last more than 10 seconds. TLESRs are part of the normal belch reflex triggered by gaseous distention of the stomach, enabling the gas trapped in the stomach to be expelled in the form of a belch. TLESRs are mediated by the nucleus tractus solitarius in the medulla, which integrates sensory information from the stomach and directs the neural circuits that produce TLESRs. Neurons with γ-aminobutyric acid B ($GABA_B$) receptors inhibit TLESRs, and the $GABA_B$ agonist baclofen can decrease their frequency.[54] Unfortunately, baclofen often causes intolerable drowsiness and other side effects, and studies on its efficacy for PPI-refractory GERD are very limited. The development of other GABA$_B$ agonists, including arbaclofen placarbil and lesogaberan was abandoned because of poor clinical efficacy.[55,56]

Alginates

When alginates come into contact with gastric acid, they precipitate into a gel that forms a "raft" that floats on top of the gastric contents. This raft poses a mechanical barrier that displaces the postprandial acid pocket (a layer of strong, unbuffered gastric acid that forms at the gastroesophageal junction after meals) distally into the stomach and out of the esophagus. Alginates seem to be more effective than placebo and antacids for treating GERD symptoms,[57] and limited data suggest that adding alginates to PPI therapy might provide better control of GERD symptoms than PPIs alone in patients with NERD.[58]

Adding an H$_2$ Receptor Antagonist at Bedtime to Proton Pump Inhibitor Therapy

Studies using gastric pH monitoring have shown that some 70% to 80% of individuals treated with twice-daily PPIs experience nocturnal gastric acid breakthrough, defined as a fall in gastric pH below 4 for more than 1 hour at night.[59] Nocturnal gastric acid breakthrough provides the opportunity for acid reflux during sleep in patients with GERD who take PPIs. Nocturnal gastric acid breakthrough seems to be largely a histamine-driven event, and short-term studies have shown that nocturnal gastric pH can be maintained above 4 by adding a bedtime dose of an H$_2$RA.[60] However, the clinical importance of nocturnal gastric acid breakthrough is not clear, and tachyphylaxis to the antisecretory effect of H$_2$RAs develops quickly.[61] Presently, few data support the clinical efficacy of adding an H$_2$RA at bedtime for patients with persistent GERD symptoms on PPI therapy.[62]

Potassium-Competitive Acid Blockers

Like PPIs, the potassium-competitive acid blockers (P-CABs) block gastric acid production by inhibiting the H$^+$, K$^+$-ATPase of the gastric parietal cell. Unlike PPIs, the P-CABs are not degraded by gastric acid and so require no enteric coating that would delay their absorption, and P-CABs are active drugs, not prodrugs. Also unlike PPIs, the P-CABs bind ionically (not covalently) to proton pumps, and since they will bind both active and inactive proton pumps they do not have to be dosed around meals. Thus, P-CABs can block gastric acid secretion more quickly than PPIs, and perhaps even more effectively than PPIs.[63] However, P-CABs are not presently available for widespread clinical use outside of Japan. Japanese studies on the P-CAB vonoprazan have demonstrated its efficacy in healing erosive esophagitis not healed by conventional-dose PPIs.[64] However, despite their theoretic advantages over PPIs, it is not clear that P-CABs are any more effective than PPIs for treating GERD in Western patients. If P-CABs become available for use in Western countries, it is anticipated that they might be especially useful for patients with persistently abnormal esophageal acid exposure on double-dose PPI therapy.

Neuromodulators

Neuromodulators, such as tricyclic antidepressants, trazadone, and selective serotonin reuptake inhibitors are thought to dull visceral hypersensitivity through effects on central nervous system pain-processing pathways. For patients with reflux hypersensitivity and functional heartburn, neuromodulators used in dosages that allegedly do not alter mood seem to have some efficacy in relieving heartburn.[65–67] However, 1 randomized controlled trial found that imipramine did not relieve symptoms any more effectively than placebo in these patients, although there were benefits of imipramine for improving quality of life.[68] Unfortunately, the neuromodulators often have intolerable and sometimes dangerous side effects, and studies on their efficacy for PPI-refractory heartburn are few and of short duration.

Cognitive Behavioral Therapy

Limited data suggest that cognitive behavioral therapy can be an effective treatment for patients with functional heartburn and reflux hypersensitivity.[69] A health psychologist with specialization in gastroenterology can be a valuable asset in patient management but, unfortunately, the availability of such therapists is limited.

Antireflux Procedures

Unlike PPIs, which target gastric acid but do nothing to correct the underlying reflux diathesis, antireflux procedures (surgical and endoscopic) are designed to create a barrier to the reflux of all gastric contents. Among all the antireflux procedures, fundoplication is considered the gold standard for its efficacy in improving the physiologic parameters of GERD, such as LES pressure and esophageal acid exposure time.[70] In principle, fundoplication should be an effective treatment for any PPI-refractory GERD symptom that is reflux related. In practice, however, patients with "GERD symptoms" that do not respond to PPIs often do not respond to surgery either.[71] When surgery fails to relieve PPI-refractory GERD symptoms, the failure is often one of poor patient choice rather than failure of the operation to control reflux. Functional disorders are a more common cause of PPI-refractory heartburn than persistent GERD, and surgery is unlikely to benefit a patient with functional complaints.[20,21] When considering surgery for patients with PPI-refractory heartburn, a thorough preoperative workup is required to exclude the functional and non-GERD organic disorders that might cause the symptom, and to ensure that the heartburn is indeed reflux related.

Laparoscopic fundoplication is an effective and reasonably safe procedure for carefully selected patients with PPI-refractory heartburn that is reflux related. Modern laparoscopic antireflux surgery has a short-term complication rate (infection, bleeding, esophageal perforation) of approximately 4%, a very low surgical mortality rate, and a GERD recurrence rate of approximately 18% within 5 years postoperatively.[72] Fundoplication can be complicated by dysphagia and by an inability to belch and vomit, and occasionally by other troublesome symptoms.

Magnetic sphincter augmentation (MSA) was developed as a less invasive and more readily reversible GERD treatment than fundoplication. In MSA, the surgeon fastens a bracelet of magnetic beads (the LINX Reflux Management System) around the distal esophagus to bolster the LES and prevent reflux. MSA seems to be an effective and durable therapy in carefully selected patients with GERD with symptoms incompletely controlled by PPIs, usually those with small hiatal hernias (<3 cm), mild or no reflux esophagitis, and documented abnormal esophageal acid exposure.[73] For patients in whom regurgitation is the predominant PPI-refractory symptom, a recent randomized trial has established the unequivocal superiority of MSA over twice-daily PPIs.[74]

Many endoscopic therapies for GERD have been developed, and most of the devices have been removed from the marketplace because of concerns regarding safety and efficacy. Presently, the only endoscopic GERD treatments still widely available are radiofrequency antireflux treatment (Stretta) and TIF. The role of Stretta is particularly controversial. Some data suggest that Stretta can be effective in carefully selected patients with GERD who are dissatisfied with PPI therapy.[75] However, a recent systematic review and meta-analysis concluded that Stretta does not significantly alter physiologic parameters, such as esophageal acid exposure and LES pressure, does not reliably enable patients to stop PPIs, and does not significantly improve health-related quality of life.[76] Randomized trials have shown that TIF is effective for treating troublesome regurgitation, at least in the short term.[77,78] Unfortunately, TIF seems to break down over time, and its long-term benefit in controlling GERD is not established and highly questionable.[70]

A system for GERD treatment via electrical stimulation of the LES is being studied. This system uses a pacemaker-like generator (EndoStim) that is implanted in the abdominal wall and connected through a cable to a pair of electrodes that are sutured to the LES muscle. Preliminary data have shown some short-term efficacy for this technique, but complications, including bowel injury during implantation and erosion of the electrode leads have been reported.[79] The device presently is not widely available, and it is not yet clear precisely how it works to control GERD. Further studies are needed before it can be recommended for clinical use.

MANAGEMENT OF PATIENTS WITH HEARTBURN REFRACTORY TO PROTON PUMP INHIBITOR THERAPY

Fig. 1 outlines an approach to the management of patients with heartburn refractory to PPI therapy. The first step is to obtain a careful medical history to confirm that the patient truly has heartburn, and to identify warning symptoms, such as dysphagia, weight loss, and gastrointestinal bleeding that might require expedited evaluation. The history might also provide clues regarding the presence of extraesophageal disease (eg, heart, pancreaticobiliary) that might be causing the heartburn sensation, and that might require urgent evaluation.

Many patients referred to gastroenterologists for PPI-refractory heartburn already are taking PPIs in high dosage, but they often are taking the PPIs incorrectly. A trial of twice-daily PPI therapy should be implemented with explicit instruction to take the PPIs 30 to 60 minutes before breakfast and dinner. Consideration can also be given to switching PPIs, especially for patients already on twice-daily PPI treatment, and for those taking pantoprazole, which is the least potent of the available PPIs for gastric acid suppression. These steps can be taken before proceeding with invasive tests. If heartburn does not improve after 4 to 8 weeks of this PPI trial, further workup is required.

I recommend stopping PPIs if possible (some patients will not tolerate a period off PPIs) for 3 to 4 weeks before proceeding to endoscopic examination. Although the PPIs are stopped in anticipation of endoscopy, consideration can be given to performing esophageal pH monitoring. The utility of pH monitoring at this point in the workup is controversial.[65] The major argument for performing it here is that a normal esophageal pH monitoring study off PPIs eliminates GERD as a diagnostic concern, and thus should direct further diagnostic and therapeutic efforts at non-GERD disorders. The counterargument is that many patients will have an abnormal pH monitoring study off PPIs and, although this establishes the presence of GERD, it does not establish that GERD is the cause of the PPI-refractory heartburn and it does not explain why the patients have not responded to PPIs. The physician's assessment of the pretest probability for GERD can be used to guide the choice of whether or not to perform esophageal pH monitoring off PPIs. If the physician determines that there is a high pretest probability for GERD or that other tests already have established that the patient has GERD (eg, a previous endoscopy showed long-segment Barrett's esophagus or severe reflux esophagitis), then pH monitoring off PPIs is unlikely to provide useful

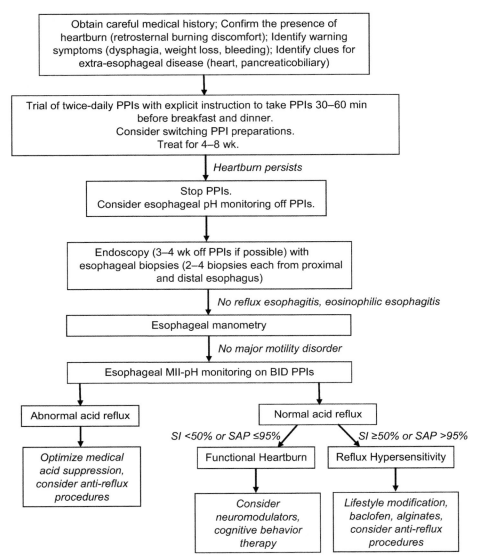

Fig. 1. Approach to the management of patients with heartburn refractory to PPI therapy.

information. Conversely, if the pretest probability for GERD is low (eg, the heartburn description is questionable or there has been no response whatsoever to PPIs), then esophageal pH monitoring can be helpful for guiding further evaluation and treatment.

It is important that PPIs be stopped for 3 to 4 if possible before performing diagnostic endoscopy. PPIs can eliminate the endoscopic and histologic signs of EoE, and so an endoscopy performed with a patient on PPI therapy cannot rule out EoE. PPIs also can eliminate all endoscopic signs of GERD, and so stopping PPIs might establish the presence of reflux esophagitis. Although it is common for physicians to make a diagnosis of NERD when endoscopy for heartburn shows no reflux esophagitis, that diagnosis is inappropriate unless PPIs were stopped. Irrespective of the appearance of the esophagus, 2 to 4 biopsies should be taken from both the proximal and distal esophagus to look for EoE.

If endoscopy shows no evidence of EoE or reflux esophagitis, esophageal manometry is performed to identify motility abnormalities, such as achalasia or distal esophageal spasm that can cause the symptom of heartburn. If there is no major motility disorder, then esophageal MII-pH monitoring is performed with the patient on twice-daily PPIs. If there is persistent abnormal acid reflux, then therapy can be focused on optimizing medical acid suppression or on controlling reflux with an antireflux procedure. If there is normal acid reflux and the SI and/or SAP are negative (ie, SI <50%, SAP ≤95%), then the patient has functional heartburn, which might be treated with neuromodulators or with cognitive behavior therapy. If the SI and/or SAP are positive (ie, SI ≥50%, SAP >95%) in the patient with normal acid reflux, then reflux hypersensitivity is diagnosed. Patients with reflux hypersensitivity can be treated with antireflux lifestyle modifications, baclofen and alginates. Antireflux procedures, such as fundoplication and MSA can be recommended in highly selected patients.

DISCLOSURE

S.J. Spechler has served as a consultant for Takeda Pharmaceuticals, Frazier Life Sciences, Phathom Pharmaceuticals, and Ironwood Pharmaceuticals, and receives royalties as an author for UpToDate.

REFERENCES

1. Gyawali CP, Fass R. Management of gastroesophageal reflux disease. Gastroenterology 2018;154:302–18.
2. Kahrilas PJ, Shaheen NJ, Vaezi MF, American Gastroenterological Association Institute, Clinical Practice and Quality Management Committee. American Gastroenterological Association Institute technical review on the management of gastroesophageal reflux disease. Gastroenterology 2008;135:1392–413.
3. Sifrim D, Zerbib F. Diagnosis and management of patients with reflux symptoms refractory to proton pump inhibitors. Gut 2012;61:1340–54.
4. Yadlapati R, DeLay K. Proton pump inhibitor-refractory gastroesophageal reflux disease. Med Clin North Am 2019;103:15–27.
5. Katz PO, Gerson LB, Vela MF. Guidelines for the diagnosis and management of gastroesophageal reflux disease. Am J Gastroenterol 2013;108:308–28.
6. Fass R, Sifrim D. Management of heartburn not responding to proton pump inhibitors. Gut 2009;58:295–309.
7. Gyawali CP, Kahrilas PJ, Savarino E, et al. Modern diagnosis of GERD: the Lyon Consensus. Gut 2018;67:1351–62.
8. Bytzer P, Jones R, Vakil N, et al. Limited ability of the proton-pump inhibitor test to identify patients with gastroesophageal reflux disease. Clin Gastroenterol Hepatol 2012;10:1360–6.
9. Kahrilas PJ, Hughes N, Howden CW. Response of unexplained chest pain to proton pump inhibitor treatment in patients with and without objective evidence of gastro-oesophageal reflux disease. Gut 2011;60:1473–8.
10. Hom C, Vaezi MF. Extraesophageal manifestations of gastroesophageal reflux disease. Gastroenterol Clin North Am 2013;42:71–91.

11. Chang AB, Lasserson TJ, Gaffney J, et al. Gastro-oesophageal reflux treatment for prolonged non-specific cough in children and adults. Cochrane Database Syst Rev 2011;(1):CD004823.

12. Vaezi MF, Richter JE, Stasney CR, et al. Treatment of chronic posterior laryngitis with esomeprazole. Laryngoscope 2006;116:254–60.

13. Spantideas N, Drosou E, Bougea A, et al. Proton pump inhibitors for the treatment of laryngopharyngeal reflux. A systematic review. J Voice 2019 [pii:S0892-1997(19)30102-X].

14. Boeckxstaens G, El-Serag HB, Smout AJ, et al. Symptomatic reflux disease: the present, the past and the future. Gut 2014;63:1185–93.

15. Kahrilas PJ, Boeckxstaens G, Smout AJ. Management of the patient with incomplete response to PPI therapy. Best Pract Res Clin Gastroenterol 2013;27:401–14.

16. Lechien JR, Akst LM, Hamdan AL, et al. Evaluation and management of laryngopharyngeal reflux disease: state of the art review. Otolaryngol Head Neck Surg 2019;160:762–82.

17. Milstein CF, Charbel S, Hicks DM, et al. Prevalence of laryngeal irritation signs associated with reflux in asymptomatic volunteers: impact of endoscopic technique (rigid vs. flexible laryngoscope). Laryngoscope 2005;115:2256–61.

18. Shin JM, Sachs G. Pharmacology of proton pump inhibitors. Curr Gastroenterol Rep 2008;10:528–34.

19. Gunaratnam NT, Jessup TP, Inadomi J, et al. Sub-optimal proton pump inhibitor dosing is prevalent in patients with poorly controlled gastro-oesophageal reflux disease. Aliment Pharmacol Ther 2006;23:1473–7.

20. Spechler SJ, Lee RH, Smith BR, et al. A VA cooperative, randomized trial of medical and surgical treatments for patients with heartburn that is refractory to proton pump inhibitors. Gastroenterology 2018;154(Supplement 1):S-1–29.

21. Spechler SJ, Lee RH, Smith BR, et al. Characterization of conditions underlying heartburn refractory to proton pump inhibitors (PPIs) in a VA cooperative study of medical and surgical treatments for PPI-refractory heartburn. Gastroenterology 2018;154(Supplement 1). S-101–102.

22. Kirchheiner J, Glatt S, Fuhr U, et al. Relative potency of proton-pump inhibitors-comparison of effects on intragastric pH. Eur J Clin Pharmacol 2009;65:19–31.

23. Graham DY, Tansel A. Interchangeable use of proton pump inhibitors based on relative potency. Clin Gastroenterol Hepatol 2018;16:800–8.

24. Katz PO, Koch FK, Ballard ED, et al. Comparison of the effects of immediate-release omeprazole oral suspension, delayed-release lansoprazole capsules and delayed-release esomeprazole capsules on nocturnal gastric acidity after bedtime dosing in patients with night-time GERD symptoms. Aliment Pharmacol Ther 2007;25(2):197–205.

25. Vakil N, van Zanten SV, Kahrilas P, et al, Global Consensus Group. The Montreal definition and classification of gastroesophageal reflux disease: a global evidence-based consensus. Am J Gastroenterol 2006;101:1900–20.

26. Spechler SJ, Jain SK, Tendler DA, et al. Racial differences in the frequency of symptoms and complications of gastro-oesophageal reflux disease. Aliment Pharmacol Ther 2002;16:1795–800.

27. Fass R, Naliboff B, Higa L, et al. Differential effect of long-term esophageal acid exposure on mechanosensitivity and chemosensitivity in humans. Gastroenterology 1998;115:1363–73.

28. Spechler SJ. Surgery for gastroesophageal reflux disease: esophageal impedance to progress? Clin Gastroenterol Hepatol 2009;7:1264–5.

29. Aziz Q, Fass R, Gyawali CP, et al. Functional esophageal disorders. Gastroenterology 2016;150:1368–79.
30. Spechler SJ, Sharma P, Traxler B, et al. Gastric and esophageal pH in patients with Barrett's esophagus treated with three esomeprazole dosages: a randomized, double-blind, crossover trial. Am J Gastroenterol 2006;101:1964–71.
31. Gerson LB, Boparai V, Ullah N, et al. Oesophageal and gastric pH profiles in patients with gastro-oesophageal reflux disease and Barrett's oesophagus treated with proton pump inhibitors. Aliment Pharmacol Ther 2004;20(6):637–43.
32. Charbel S, Khandwala F, Vaezi MF. The role of esophageal pH monitoring in symptomatic patients on PPI therapy. Am J Gastroenterol 2005;100:283–9.
33. Bautista JM, Wong WM, Pulliam G, et al. The value of ambulatory 24 hr esophageal pH monitoring in clinical practice in patients who were referred with persistent gastroesophageal reflux disease (GERD)-related symptoms while on standard dose anti-reflux medications. Dig Dis Sci 2005;50:1909–15.
34. Sifrim D, Mittal R, Fass R, et al. Review article: acidity and volume of the refluxate in the genesis of gastro-oesophageal reflux disease symptoms. Aliment Pharmacol Ther 2007;25:1003–17.
35. Mittal RK, Liu J, Puckett JL, et al. Sensory and motor function of the esophagus: lessons from ultrasound imaging. Gastroenterology 2005;128:487–97.
36. Wiener GJ, Richter JE, Copper JB, et al. The symptom index: a clinically important parameter of ambulatory 24-hour esophageal pH monitoring. Am J Gastroenterol 1988;83:358–61.
37. Weusten BL, Roelofs JM, Akkermans LM, et al. The symptom-association probability: an improved method for symptom analysis of 24-hour esophageal pH data. Gastroenterology 1994;107:1741–5.
38. Kahrilas PJ. When proton pump inhibitors fail. Clin Gastroenterol Hepatol 2008; 6(5):482–3.
39. Choksi Y, Slaughter JC, Sharda R, et al. Symptom association probability does not reliably distinguish functional heartburn from reflux hypersensitivity. Aliment Pharmacol Ther 2018;47(7):958–65.
40. Cheng E, Souza RF, Spechler SJ. Eosinophilic esophagitis: interactions with gastroesophageal reflux disease. Gastroenterol Clin North Am 2014;43:243–56.
41. Liacouras CA, Furuta GT, Hirano I, et al. Eosinophilic esophagitis: updated consensus recommendations for children and adults. J Allergy Clin Immunol 2011;128:3–20.
42. Dellon ES, Liacouras CA, Molina-Infante J, et al. Updated international consensus diagnostic criteria for eosinophilic esophagitis: proceedings of the AGREE conference. Gastroenterology 2018;155:1022–33.
43. Odiase E, Schwartz A, Souza RF, et al. New eosinophilic esophagitis concepts call for change in proton pump inhibitor management before diagnostic endoscopy. Gastroenterology 2018;154:1217–21.
44. Spechler SJ, Souza RF, Rosenberg SJ, et al. Heartburn in patients with achalasia. Gut 1995;37:305–8.
45. Smart HL, Foster PN, Evans DF, et al. Twenty four hour oesophageal acidity in achalasia before and after pneumatic dilatation. Gut 1987;28:883–7.
46. Kessing BF, Bredenoord AJ, Smout AJPM. Erroneous diagnosis of gastroesophageal reflux disease in achalasia. Clin Gastroenterol Hepatol 2011;9:1020–4.
47. Chang P, Friedenberg F. Obesity and GERD. Gastroenterol Clin North Am 2014; 43:161–73.

48. Teragawa H, Oshita C, Ueda T. History of gastroesophageal reflux disease in patients with suspected coronary artery disease. Heart Vessels 2019;34(10): 1631–8.

49. Bösner S, Haasenritter J, Becker A, et al. Heartburn or angina? Differentiating gastrointestinal disease in primary care patients presenting with chest pain: a cross sectional diagnostic study. Int Arch Med 2009;2:40.

50. Schmulson MJ, Drossman DA. What is new in Rome IV. J Neurogastroenterol Motil 2017;23:151–63.

51. Vela MF, Camacho-Lobato L, Srinivasan R, et al. Simultaneous intraesophageal impedance and pH measurement of acid and nonacid gastroesophageal reflux: effect of omeprazole. Gastroenterology 2001;120:1599–606.

52. Kahrilas PJ, Jonsson A, Denison H, et al. Regurgitation is less responsive to acid suppression than heartburn in patients with gastroesophageal reflux disease. Clin Gastroenterol Hepatol 2012;10:612–9.

53. Kessing BF, Conchillo JM, Bredenoord AJ, et al. Review article: the clinical relevance of transient lower oesophageal sphincter relaxations in gastro-oesophageal reflux disease. Aliment Pharmacol Ther 2011;33:650–61.

54. Li S, Shi S, Chen F, et al. The effects of baclofen for the treatment of gastroesophageal reflux disease: a meta-analysis of randomized controlled trials. Gastroenterol Res Pract 2014;2014:307805.

55. Vakil NB, Huff FJ, Bian A, et al. Arbaclofen placarbil in GERD: a randomized, double-blind, placebo-controlled study. Am J Gastroenterol 2011;106:1427–38.

56. Boeckxstaens GE, Beaumont H, Hatlebakk JG, et al. A novel reflux inhibitor lesogaberan (AZD3355) as add-on treatment in patients with GORD with persistent reflux symptoms despite proton pump inhibitor therapy: a randomised placebo-controlled trial. Gut 2011;60:1182–8.

57. Leiman DA, Riff BP, Morgan S, et al. Alginate therapy is effective treatment for GERD symptoms: a systematic review and meta-analysis. Dis Esophagus 2017;30:1–9.

58. Manabe N, Haruma K, Ito M, et al. Efficacy of adding sodium alginate to omeprazole in patients with nonerosive reflux disease: a randomized clinical trial. Dis Esophagus 2012;25:373–80.

59. Katz PO, Anderson C, Khoury R, et al. Gastro-oesophageal reflux associated with nocturnal gastric acid breakthrough on proton pump inhibitors. Aliment Pharmacol Ther 1998;12:1231–4.

60. Peghini PL, Katz PO, Castell DO. Ranitidine controls nocturnal gastric acid breakthrough on omeprazole: a controlled study in normal subjects. Gastroenterology 1998;115:1335–9.

61. Fackler WK, Ours TM, Vaezi MF, et al. Long-term effect of H2RA therapy on nocturnal gastric acid breakthrough. Gastroenterology 2002;122:625–32.

62. Wang Y, Pan T, Wang Q, et al. Additional bedtime H2-receptor antagonist for the control of nocturnal gastric acid breakthrough. Cochrane Database Syst Rev 2009;(4):CD004275.

63. Hunt RH, Scarpignato C. Potassium-competitive acid blockers (P-CABs): are they finally ready for prime time in acid-related disease? Clin Transl Gastroenterol 2015;6:e119.

64. Tanabe T, Hoshino S, Kawami N, et al. Efficacy of long-term maintenance therapy with 10-mg vonoprazan for proton pump inhibitor-resistant reflux esophagitis. Esophagus 2019;16(4):377–81.

65. Weijenborg PW, de Schepper HS, Smout AJ, et al. Effects of antidepressants in patients with functional esophageal disorders or gastroesophageal reflux disease: a systematic review. Clin Gastroenterol Hepatol 2015;13:251–9.

66. Drossman DA, Tack J, Ford AC, et al. Neuromodulators for functional gastrointestinal disorders (disorders of gut-brain interaction): a Rome Foundation Working Team Report. Gastroenterology 2018;154:1140–71.

67. Viazis N, Keyoglou A, Kanellopoulos AK, et al. Selective serotonin reuptake inhibitors for the treatment of hypersensitive esophagus: a randomized, double-blind, placebo-controlled study. Am J Gastroenterol 2012;107:1662–7.

68. Limsrivilai J, Charatcharoenwitthaya P, Pausawasdi N, et al. Imipramine for treatment of esophageal hypersensitivity and functional heartburn: a randomized placebo-controlled trial. Am J Gastroenterol 2016;111:217–24.

69. Riehl ME, Kinsinger S, Kahrilas PJ, et al. Role of a health psychologist in the management of functional esophageal complaints. Dis Esophagus 2015;28:428–36.

70. Richter JE, Kumar A, Lipka S, et al. Efficacy of laparoscopic Nissen fundoplication vs transoral incisionless fundoplication or proton pump inhibitors in patients with gastroesophageal reflux disease: a systematic review and network meta-analysis. Gastroenterology 2018;154:1298–308.

71. Morgenthal CB, Lin E, Shane MD, et al. Who will fail laparoscopic Nissen fundoplication? Preoperative prediction of long-term outcomes. Surg Endosc 2007;21:1978–84.

72. Maret-Ouda J, Wahlin K, El-Serag HB, et al. Association between laparoscopic antireflux surgery and recurrence of gastroesophageal reflux. JAMA 2017;318:939–46.

73. Saino G, Bonavina L, Lipham JC, et al. Magnetic sphincter augmentation for gastroesophageal reflux at 5 years: final results of a pilot study show long-term acid reduction and symptom improvement. J Laparoendosc Adv Surg Tech A 2015;25:787–92.

74. Bell R, Lipham J, Louie B, et al. Laparoscopic magnetic sphincter augmentation versus double-dose proton pump inhibitors for management of moderate-to-severe regurgitation in GERD: a randomized controlled trial. Gastrointest Endosc 2019;89:14–22.

75. Viswanath Y, Maguire N, Obuobi RB, et al. Endoscopic day case antireflux radiofrequency (Stretta) therapy improves quality of life and reduce proton pump inhibitor (PPI) dependency in patients with gastro-oesophageal reflux disease: a prospective study from a UK tertiary centre. Frontline Gastroenterol 2019;10:113–9.

76. Lipka S, Kumar A, Richter JE. No evidence for efficacy of radiofrequency ablation for treatment of gastroesophageal reflux disease: a systematic review and meta-analysis. Clin Gastroenterol Hepatol 2015;13:1058–67.

77. Hunter JG, Kahrilas PJ, Bell RC, et al. Efficacy of transoral fundoplication vs omeprazole for treatment of regurgitation in a randomized controlled trial. Gastroenterology 2015;148:324–33.

78. Trad KS, Barnes WE, Simoni G, et al. Transoral incisionless fundoplication effective in eliminating GERD symptoms in partial responders to proton pump inhibitor therapy at 6 months: the TEMPO Randomized Clinical Trial. Surg Innov 2015;22:26–40.

79. Kappelle WF, Bredenoord AJ, Conchillo JM, et al. Electrical stimulation therapy of the lower oesophageal sphincter for refractory gastro-oesophageal reflux disease - interim results of an international multicentre trial. Aliment Pharmacol Ther 2015;42:614–25.

Laryngopharyngeal Reflux and Atypical Gastroesophageal Reflux Disease

Caroline M. Barrett, MD[a], Dhyanesh Patel, MD[b],*,
Michael F. Vaezi, MD, PhD[b]

KEYWORDS

• Extraesophageal reflux disease • Laryngopharyngeal reflux • Chronic cough

KEY POINTS

• Extraesophageal reflux syndromes represent a significant economic health care burden in the United States owing to delay in recognition of the diagnosis, lack of a gold standard diagnostic test, and lack of effective therapies.

• The reflex theory describes the most likely underlying pathophysiology. There is emerging evidence for the role of autonomic nerve dysfunction and neuronal hyperresponsiveness in disease.

• Current diagnostic modalities, specifically laryngoscopy, esophagogastroduodenoscopy, ambulatory pH, and pH-impedance monitoring, are limited by poor sensitivity and specificity and high interrater variability for diagnosis of laryngopharyngeal reflux.

• Newer biomarkers and mucosal integrity testing show promise for diagnosis, but further controlled trials are needed.

• There is a lack of clear evidence in support of the use of proton pump inhibitors or for the role of antireflux surgery in patients with laryngopharyngeal reflux.

INTRODUCTION

Gastroesophageal reflux disease (GERD) affects an estimated 18% to 28% of the population in the United States, making it the most prevalent gastrointestinal disorder in the country.[1] GERD is a spectrum of disease that can be divided into 2 classes: esophageal syndromes (typical GERD), characterized by heartburn and regurgitation; and extraesophageal syndromes (atypical GERD), which can manifest with various other symptoms, such as hoarseness, chronic cough, and globus pharyngeus.[2]

[a] Department of Internal Medicine, Vanderbilt University Medical Center, 719 Thompson Lane, Suite 20400, Nashville, TN 37204, USA; [b] Division of Gastroenterology, Hepatology and Nutrition, Vanderbilt University Medical Center, 1301 Medical Center Drive, TVC # 1660, Nashville, TN 37232, USA
* Corresponding author.
E-mail address: Dan.patel@vumc.org

Gastrointest Endoscopy Clin N Am 30 (2020) 361–376
https://doi.org/10.1016/j.giec.2019.12.004

The mean direct cost to diagnose and treat a patient with typical GERD in the first year of evaluation is $971 per patient.[3] However, the evaluation and treatment of extraesophageal reflux (EER) has averaged $5438 per patient in the first year.[3] When these numbers are extrapolated to estimate total economic burden among the US population, the annual national expenditures for the treatment of GERD range from $9.3 billion[4] to $12.1 billion,[5] making the estimated annual cost of EER 5 times that at $50 billion,[3] as outlined in **Fig. 1**. The higher health care burden of EER can be attributed to delay in recognition of the diagnosis, lack of a gold standard diagnostic test, lack of effective treatment, and the widespread use of proton pump inhibitors (PPIs).[3]

Diagnosis of laryngopharyngeal reflux (LPR), a subtype of extraesophageal reflux, proves more difficult than typical GERD because of the lack of typical symptoms of heartburn and regurgitation and the attribution of many varied symptoms to the disease (**Table 1**). It is estimated to account for 10% of all ear, nose, and throat (ENT) clinic patients and 50% of patients with voice complaints.[6] LPR is characterized most commonly by dysphonia (71%), chronic cough (51%), globus pharyngeus (47%), and recurrent throat clearing (42%).[6] Despite the lack of a gold standard diagnostic method, the diagnosis of EER is a common one made by primary care physicians, otolaryngologists, allergists, and gastroenterologists and has been the subject of much research.[7]

This article reviews important clinical articles in the gastroenterology literature, examining the pathophysiology, diagnosis, and treatment options for extraesophageal GERD and laryngopharyngeal reflux.

PATHOPHYSIOLOGY

Controversy exists over the underlying physiologic mechanism linking esophageal reflux to extraesophageal symptoms. The reflux theory postulates that esophagopharyngeal reflux through microaspiration of acid, bile acids, and pepsin results in direct injury to the larynx.[8] An alternative mechanism, the reflex theory, proposes that acidification of the distal esophagus induces laryngeal symptoms through a vagally mediated reflex.[9,10] In examining the pathophysiology of reflux-induced cough, patients with positive symptom association probability for reflux preceding cough have no greater esophageal exposure to reflux but do have a more sensitive cough reflex, suggesting a sensitized central mechanism facilitating reflux-induced cough.[11] Measurements of pepsin concentration in sputum and bronchoalveolar lavage samples have revealed that microaspiration into the airways and proximal gastroesophageal reflux have a limited role in contributing to cough in patients with unselected chronic cough and confirmed GERD.[12] Furthermore, in a study examining the determinants of reflux-induced cough, the acidity of the refluxate was not relevant in distinguishing reflux

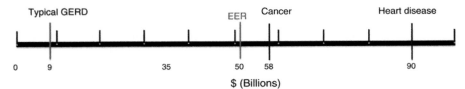

Fig. 1. Estimated economic health care burden of EER compared with typical GERD, cancer, and heart disease. (*From* Francis DO, Rymer JA, Slaughter JC, et al. High economic burden of caring for patients with suspected extraesophageal reflux. *Am J Gastroenterol.* 2013;108(6):905-911; with permission.)

Table 1
Laryngopharyngeal and other symptoms of extraesophageal reflux

Laryngopharyngeal	Respiratory	Other
Dysphonia	Chronic cough	Postnasal drip
Hoarseness	Apnea	Atypical chest pain
Sore throat	Asthma	Dental erosions
Globus pharyngeus	Chronic obstructive pulmonary disease	Sinusitis
Throat clearing	Recurrent pneumonia	Otitis media
Laryngospasm	Pulmonary fibrosis	
Laryngeal cancer	Lung transplant rejection	
Pharyngitis		
Laryngitis		

episodes that were or were not related to cough.[13] However, a larger volume of refluxate and longer esophageal exposure time to reflux were more associated with cough. Reflux episodes only reaching the distal esophagus were still able to trigger cough, and most reflux episodes that did reach the proximal esophagus did not result in cough, supporting the reflex rather than reflux theory.[13]

Hypersensitivity Syndrome

Recently, Wang and colleagues[14] showed that patients with laryngopharyngeal reflux disease have less vagal nerve function and more sympathetic nerve activity compared with controls, suggesting the role of autonomic nerve dysfunction in the pathogenesis of LPR. The investigators conclude that autonomic nerve dysfunction in the esophagus leads to dysregulation of peristalsis and function of both lower and upper esophageal sphincters. The severity of LPR was correlated with the degree of autonomic nerve dysfunction as well.[14] This finding further strengthens the theory that most of these patients might have an abnormality of the neuronal pathways controlling symptoms such as cough and that identified causes (including asthma, reflux, and postnasal drip) might act as triggers only in the context of neuronal hypersensitivity.[15] A study involving inhalation of capsaicin (an irritant aerosol) showed that patients with chronic cough were twice as likely to have a cough response compared with healthy controls.[16] This concept of neuronal hyperresponsiveness is also consistent clinically because patients with laryngeal symptoms often report sensation of throat irritation, irresistible urge to cough, and coughing triggered by low levels of environmental changes (dust, perfumes, changes in temperature/humidity), and even physical stimulation (singing and eating).[17,18] Thus, there is now a newer focus on developing therapeutic options that target specific neuronal receptors in both the peripheral and the central nervous system (such as P2X3,[19] and transient receptor potential [TRP] vanilloid 1 [TRPA1], vanilloid 4 [TRPV4], and ankyrin 1 [TRPA1]).[20] In a recent randomized controlled trial in patients with refractory chronic cough, P2X3 antagonist treatment was associated with a 75% greater reduction in cough counts compared with baseline.[19] The study adds further understanding to the complicated pathophysiology of this disease and may have implications for future treatment strategies.

DIAGNOSTIC MODALITIES

The diagnosis of laryngopharyngeal reflux proves to be more difficult than typical GERD because of the lack of a definitive testing methodology.[21] There is much uncertainty on how best to diagnose LPR, with most testing methodologies, such as laryngoscopy, upper endoscopy, and pH monitoring, all showing poor sensitivity in detecting in whom reflux may be the cause of laryngeal symptoms. There are currently no diagnostic tests that unequivocally link any extraesophageal symptoms to GERD.

Laryngoscopy

LPR is a diagnosis of exclusion, and note that other disease processes, both benign and malignant, can present with similar symptoms (**Table 2**). The first step in diagnosis should involve a careful history and physical. Malignancy of the larynx or pharynx can have an insidious course, presenting with vague symptoms of hoarseness, sore throat, and globus sensation. Furthermore, both GERD and laryngopharyngeal reflux disease have been associated with laryngeal malignancy.[22] In a systematic review and meta-analysis of 18 case-control studies, patients with reflux disease were 2.5 times more likely to also have laryngeal malignancy. Most of the studies examined the relationship between GERD and laryngeal malignancy, but, in those that studied patients with LPR, the investigators were able to conclude that patients were 3.1 times more likely to have had a diagnosis of prior laryngeal malignancy.[22] If risk factors for malignancy are identified, such as smoking, alcohol use, night sweats, and/or weight loss, then the first step in diagnosis should involve ruling out malignancy with laryngoscopy.[7] The diagnosis of EER should then be considered if there are any signs of laryngeal inflammation.[23] Laryngoscopic findings of LPR include vocal cord edema, erythema, ventricular obliteration, and pseudosulcus ovalis (**Box 1**).[24]

Laryngoscopy has been criticized for its lack of specificity, poor reliability, and high interobserver variability.[10,25] One study found that 86% of healthy volunteer subjects had hypopharynx findings that have been associated with GERD.[26] Another found that signs of posterior laryngeal irritation were present in greater

---

Table 2
Laryngopharyngeal disorders with symptoms overlapping with those attributed to extraesophageal reflux

Disorder	Symptoms
Muscle tension dysphonia	Hoarseness, globus, throat pain, dysphagia
Vocal fold paralysis/paresis	Hoarseness, cough, dysphagia, dyspnea, globus
Presbylaryngis	Hoarseness, cough, globus
Irritable larynx syndrome	Cough, globus, hoarseness
Cancer	Throat pain, hoarseness, cough, dysphagia, dyspnea, globus, ear pain
Recurrent respiratory papillomatosis	Hoarseness, cough, dyspnea, globus
Laryngotracheal stenosis	Hoarseness, dyspnea
Phonotraumatic lesion	Hoarseness
Vocal fold hemorrhage	Hoarseness
Polypoid corditis	Hoarseness, cough, globus, dyspnea
Vocal fold scarring	Hoarseness
Vocal process granuloma	Throat pain, hoarseness, cough, globus
Laryngeal candidiasis	Throat pain, hoarseness, cough, dysphagia, globus
Zenker diverticulum	Regurgitation, hoarseness, dysphagia, globus
Paradoxic vocal fold motion	Dyspnea

From Francis DO, Vaezi MF. Should the Reflex Be Reflux? Throat Symptoms and Alternative Explanations. *Clin Gastroenterol Hepatol.* 2015;13(9):1560-1566. https://doi.org/10.1016/j.cgh.2014.08.044; with permission.

Box 1
Potential laryngoscopic findings seen in extraesophageal reflux disease

Edema and hyperemia of larynx

Hyperemia and lymphoid hyperplasia of posterior pharynx

Interarytenoid changes

Granuloma

Contact ulcers

Laryngeal polyps

Reinke edema

Tumors

Subglottic stenosis

Posterior glottic stenosis

Strictures

---

than 80% of asymptomatic individuals.[27] The diagnosis of LPR based on laryngoscopic findings often leads to unnecessary treatment. A subset of patients diagnosed with LPR by symptoms and laryngoscopy who did not respond to acid suppression underwent laparoscopic Nissen fundoplication, which did not reliably improve symptoms.[28]

Because of the lack of specific findings or a validated instrument to document laryngoscopic findings, there is high interobserver variability. This variability led to the development of a standardized scoring system, the reflux finding score (RFS), by Belafsky and colleagues.[29] The tool assesses clinical severity of 8 laryngoscopic findings (subglottic edema, ventricular obliteration, erythema/hyperemia, vocal fold edema, diffuse laryngeal edema, posterior commissure hypertrophy, granuloma/granulation tissue, and excessive endolaryngeal mucus) and provides a score ranging from 0 (normal) to 26 (worst score possible). In 40 patients with LPR diagnosed by pH monitoring, there was a 95% probability of having LPR with a score greater than 7. Belafsky and colleagues[29] showed high interobserver and intraobserver reproducibility. However, further studies questioned the interrater reliability of the score.[30-32] Because of the high interobserver variability and lack of specific findings, laryngoscopy alone should not be used to diagnose EER.

Esophagogastroduodenoscopy

In performing the history and physical, the presence of more typical symptoms of GERD, such as heartburn and regurgitation, should increase the likelihood that a patient's laryngeal symptoms are caused by EER. However, most patients have atypical symptoms alone, prompting the need for further testing. Esophagogastroduodenoscopy (EGD) is of limited utility in the evaluation of suspected EER. Esophagitis is detected in up to 20% of asymptomatic patients[33] and 40% of patients with asthma.[34] Only 20% of patients with extraesophageal symptoms have endoscopic evidence of esophagitis.[35] Few patients with erosive esophagitis have extraesophageal reflux symptoms, and the presence of esophagitis does not predict response of EER-attributed symptoms to acid suppression therapy.[21]

Ambulatory pH Monitoring

Catheter-based ambulatory pH monitoring using a 24-hour transnasal double probe (simultaneous esophageal and pharyngeal) was the previous gold standard in diagnosis of GERD, but it is unreliable in patients with laryngeal symptoms.[2,10,36] Symptom association analysis is not reliable in these patients because many extraesophageal symptoms, such as hoarseness and sore throat, are not of sufficiently sudden onset to prompt patients to press the event button. Even in patients with the symptom of cough, up to 90% of cough episodes are not reported by patients, as shown by acoustic devices.[37] Catheter-based pH monitoring has been shown to have poor sensitivity (70%–80%) and specificity (false-negative 20%–50%), and is not used in clinical practice to diagnose patients with suspected LPR.[23,38,39] This finding was further supported by a systematic review of 11 studies comparing 24-hour double (pharyngeal and esophageal) pH monitoring between normal controls and patients with clinically diagnosed reflux laryngitis, which found pharyngeal reflux events in only a minority of patients with clinically diagnosed reflux laryngitis, and there was no significant difference in pharyngeal reflux events between the two groups.[40]

In an effort to address the limitations of catheter-based pH monitoring, oropharyngeal pH monitoring was developed. Restech Dx-pH (Restech Dx-pH Measurement System, Restech Corporation) is a transnasal catheter system that measures oropharyngeal pH through detection of pH in both aerosolized and liquid droplets.[41–43] Compared with a standard pH catheter in liquid and aerosolized solutions, oropharyngeal pH monitoring is more sensitive in detecting EER.[44] In an initial study in a small pediatric population with clinical suspicion of LPR, the Restech Dx-pH measurement system detected reflux in all patients who had histopathologic changes consistent with reflux.[45] However, there is concern that it may be oversensitive: in comparing oropharyngeal pH monitoring with esophageal impedance-pH monitoring, most acidic oropharyngeal events had no temporal correlation with gastroesophageal reflux events detected by esophageal impedance-pH monitoring.[46] There have been several other studies detecting discordance between oropharyngeal pH monitoring and esophageal impedance-pH monitoring.[47,48] These studies raised questions about the understanding of the pathophysiology of LPR because reflux events did not correlate with alteration in pharyngeal pH. Further, the lack of consensus on normal and abnormal values has limited the Restech Dx-pH as a diagnostic tool.[41,43,49]

Other studies have questioned the value of oropharyngeal pH monitoring in predicting response to both medical and surgical therapy.[2,50] It has predicted response to surgical intervention,[51] but there are conflicting data on its ability to predict response to PPI therapy.[50,52,53]

Combined pH and Impedance Monitoring

Combined esophageal pH-impedance monitoring is considered the gold standard in diagnosis of esophageal reflux.[54] The poor reliability of pH testing for diagnosis of LPR led some investigators to believe that nonacidic reflux may be contributing to patient symptoms. pH-impedance monitoring can assess for nonacid reflux in patients with extraesophageal reflux. Multichannel intraluminal impedance increased diagnostic yield in detecting atypical GERD compared with impedance monitoring devices alone, pH monitors, and endoscopy.[55] However, the clinical relevance of impedance-pH monitoring remains uncertain because of the lack of treatment implications for nonacidic reflux.[2] Impedance-pH monitoring in patients on PPI therapy did not predict EER symptom response after surgical fundoplication.[56] In a group of patients with EER refractory to PPI therapy, impedance testing results on PPI therapy could not be predicted from standard baseline reflux parameters. Thus, caution should be taken in the use of impedance testing among patients with extraesophageal symptoms.[57]

Novel Tests

Salivary pepsin assay is a noninvasive test that has shown promise and has generated much research in recent years. Pepsin is a gastric enzyme that is activated from pepsinogen by hydrochloric acid in the stomach, and its presence in the saliva is thought to be secondary to reflux.[58,59] The novel pepsin test (Peptest, Biomed) detects salivary pepsin at a concentration greater than or equal to 16 ng/mL.[59] Knight and colleagues[60] first suggested the use of pepsin presence in throat sputum as a sensitive and noninvasive diagnostic method for LPR. Compared with oropharyngeal pH data for detecting reflux, pepsin immunoassay was 100% sensitive and 89% specific for LPR.[60] In an initial study, however, pepsin was not detected in the saliva of any of the 93 patients with a clinical diagnosis of LPR.[61] There have been multiple studies since, and, in a systematic review of pepsin as a marker for diagnosis of LPR, 12 studies were analyzed and all but 2 found statistically significant differences in the presence of pepsin in patients with clinical suspicion or diagnosis of LPR and healthy controls.[62] Numerous studies to date have commented on the use of salivary pepsin as a diagnostic marker for LPR, but there is no consensus on sampling techniques or cutoff values for abnormal pepsin levels at which point it should be considered pathologic.[63] A recent meta-analysis of 11 studies found a pooled sensitivity of 64% and pooled specificity of 68%. The diagnostic odds ratio was 4, meaning diagnostic accuracy was not as high as previously thought.[64] Further, it has been shown to have a positive likelihood ratio of 16.4, but a negative likelihood ratio of only 0.61, causing investigators to conclude that a negative test result should be followed by further testing.[59] It is a simple, noninvasive, inexpensive, and easily reproducible diagnostic test, but its role in diagnosis has yet to be clearly established.[21]

A newer diagnostic biomarker, squamous epithelium stress protein (Sep70), has also shown promise. Sep70 is a protective epithelial protein that assists in laryngeal defense mechanisms. Depletion of Sep70 along with the presence of pepsin in the hypopharynx together may be a marker of cellular laryngeal injury caused by LPR.[65] The Sep70/pepsin ratio is significantly lower in patients with symptomatic LPR.[63] In the study by Hoppo and colleagues,[63] each of the symptomatic subgroups had lower Sep70/pepsin ratios but specifically had higher expressions of hypopharyngeal pepsin without significant differences in Sep70 expression. In a subanalysis of 17 patients who went on to have antireflux surgery, 88% had symptomatic improvement, but no differences were seen in sep70/pepsin ratios between those with and without symptom improvement. The investigators propose that the Sep70/pepsin ratio may serve as a reliable biomarker for diagnosis of LPR. However, this has been criticized because of the novel biomarker having a specificity of only 36% and the lack of correlation with symptom response after surgery.[66]

The authors have also recently developed another device that is designed to measure conductivity of the esophageal epithelium, called mucosal integrity testing (MIT). We have previously shown that MIT is able to differentiate between GERD, nonerosive reflux disease, eosinophilic esophagitis, and normal individuals based on pattern of impedance in the esophagus instantly during endoscopy.[67,68] In a prospective longitudinal cohort study, we also found that patients with primarily EER-attributed symptoms had significantly lower MIT measurements at 2 cm above the squamocolumnar junction compared with patients without evidence of acid reflux.[69] Future studies using MIT in diagnosis and predicting treatment response in patients with EER are underway.

HAs-BEER Score

An empirical trial of twice-daily PPI therapy is the current best diagnostic and therapeutic test for patients suspected to have LPR.[23] In patients who have refractory symptoms on maximal PPI therapy and normal endoscopy, the next step in evaluation includes wireless pH monitoring or multichannel intraluminal impedance with pH (MII-pH) study. American College of Gastroenterology (ACG) guidelines currently recommend testing patients with high pretest probability of GERD with MII-pH on PPI therapy and testing those with low pretest probability with pH or MII-pH off therapy. The authors recently developed a scoring system to assist clinicians in choosing the most appropriate next diagnostic test in those with suspected EER.[70] The HAs-BEER (heartburn, asthma, BMI in extra-esophageal reflux) scoring system was developed using a clinical model and can be applied to patients with persistent extraesophageal symptoms following an 8-week course of twice-daily PPI therapy. One point each is assigned for heartburn, asthma, and/or body mass index greater than 25. A score of 3 indicates high probability of reflux, and patients should undergo impedance-pH testing on therapy to evaluate for nonacidic reflux contributing to symptoms. A score of less than or equal to 2 indicates a low probability of reflux, and these patients should undergo pH testing off therapy to rule out acidic reflux as the cause of symptoms (**Fig. 2**).

MANAGEMENT
Medical Therapy

Empiric acid suppression with 2 months of a PPI is the first step in treatment of patients with suspected LPR. There have been numerous studies investigating the efficacy of PPI therapy in this cohort of patients, and there is a lack of evidence in support of its use. In a systematic review of 14 uncontrolled studies and 6 randomized controlled trials that used PPI as empiric therapy for LPR, the uncontrolled studies showed positive results, but the randomized controlled trials (RCTs) reported no statistically significant difference in changes in frequency or severity of symptoms after treatment with PPI versus placebo.[71] In a 2006 meta-analysis analyzing data from 8 RCTs, PPI resulted in a nonsignificant reduction in symptoms compared with placebo in patients with suspected GERD-related chronic laryngitis.[72] A 2015 meta-analysis including 14 RCTs with a total of 771 patients showed that PPI therapy significantly improved symptoms compared with placebo, but there was not a significant improvement in the RFSs.[73] More recently, a 2019 systematic review included 2 systematic reviews and 7 meta-analyses: 6 of the reviews/meta-analyses proved that PPI is not superior to placebo and 3 found that PPI significantly improved LPR symptoms but did not result in significant changes in laryngoscopic findings.[74] Another 2019 systematic review and meta-analysis concluded a mild superiority of PPI compared with placebo but highlighted discrepancies among many of the 72 studies in the criteria for inclusion of patients and lack of gold standard diagnostic testing in contributing to the inability to show clear evidence in favor of use of PPI.[75]

There are differences in PPI prescribing practices among physicians, and, in a prospective randomized clinical trial comparing once-daily PPI, twice-daily PPI, and twice-daily PPI plus a prokinetic agent, the 3 strategies were similarly effective in improving reflux symptom index (RSI) and RFS.[76] Overweight and obese patients had greater improvement in RFS when the prokinetic agent was added to PPI.[76] Further evidence for the use of prokinetic agents (itopride, domperidone, tegaserod, mosapride) is limited. In a systemic review including 4 prospective studies, there was a statistically significant improvement in patient symptoms with the use of prokinetics in 3 of the 4 studies, but no significant difference in laryngeal examination findings.[77] In patients who do not respond to PPI trial and have negative reflux testing off

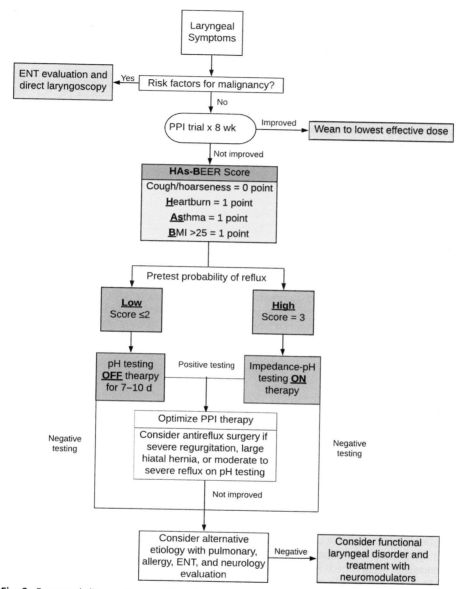

Fig. 2. Proposed diagnostic algorithm for patients with laryngeal symptoms.

therapy, GERD is unlikely to be the cause of their EER-attributed symptoms, and an alternative cause should be evaluated using a multidisciplinary approach with evaluation by ENT, allergy, neurology, and pulmonary specialists. This approach is critical to avoid unnecessary prolonged use of acid suppression in patients that do not have benefit from them.

Baclofen, a gamma-aminobutyric acid receptor type B (GABA-B) has been shown to be effective in GERD,[78] but up until recently there were no controlled studies examining its use in extraesophageal reflux disease. In a recent open-label study, 32 patients with laryngopharyngeal reflux diagnosed on 24-hour multichannel intraluminal impedance-pH who had persistent symptoms on PPI therapy were given baclofen 10 mg 3 times daily in addition to PPI 15 mg twice daily for 3 months. There was a significant improvement in RSI scores and reflux-related quality-of-life scores, and 53.1% of patients had responded at 3 months.[79]

There have been few studies examining the role of diet as therapy for LPR. In an uncontrolled study of 20 patients with pH-proven LPR and persistent symptoms on acid suppression therapy, a low-acid diet (eliminating all foods and drinks with pH<5 for 2 weeks) significantly improved symptoms (RSI) and laryngoscopic findings (RFS).[80] Diet adherence has been correlated with improvement in symptoms and finding of posterior commissure granulation severity.[81] More studies are needed to further examine the role of diet and other lifestyle modifications in the management of LPR.

Surgical Therapy

The data on surgical fundoplication are also weak, with a lack of evidence proving its benefit in the management of LPR. A review of 27 observational studies found that efficacy of antireflux surgery in LPR ranged widely, from 10% to 93%.[82] A second, more recent, systematic review is again inconclusive.[83] Thirty-four studies were reviewed, but the investigators determined they varied in inclusion/exclusion criteria, method in diagnosis of LPR, and clinical outcomes to assess efficacy of surgical fundoplication.[83] Again, lack of gold standard diagnosis limits the ability to predict for whom surgery may be of benefit. At this time, surgery is cautiously recommended for a select group of patients: those who complain of heartburn and regurgitation in addition to their primary presenting symptom, have presence of a hiatal hernia, or evidence of moderate to severe reflux at baseline off PPI therapy with continued reflux on PPI therapy.[21,56]

Novel Treatments

A novel treatment device, the upper esophageal sphincter assist device (UESAD), applies 20 to 30 mm Hg of cricoid pressure, and in turn increases the upper esophageal sphincter intraluminal pressure.[84] In a pilot study assessing the clinical efficacy of the UESAD, there was significant symptomatic improvement with use of the device, and symptom improvement was associated with reduction in salivary pepsin level. Further, all of the patients stated they would continue to use the device, and 93% of them said that they would recommend it to others.[85]

Treatment of laryngopharyngeal reflux continues to prove challenging because of variable response to PPI therapy and lack of conclusive evidence to support both the use of PPI, the best medical treatment at this time, and surgical fundoplication. If patients have negative pH testing results off PPI therapy and other causes of laryngeal symptoms have been eliminated, then a functional laryngeal disorder could be considered.[23] Laryngeal hypersensitivity may contribute to the lack of response to PPI therapy, similarly to the role that hypersensitive esophagus plays in esophageal reflux PPI nonresponders.[50,86] Neuromodulators are the mainstay of treatment in this group of patients, with most studies focusing on treatment of chronic cough as the presenting symptom. One double-blind, placebo-controlled, randomized controlled trial in patients with chronic cough for longer than 8 weeks noted significant improvement in patients that received gabapentin (up to 1800 mg/d) compared with placebo for 8 weeks, with number need to treat of 3.5.[87] This finding has led to the most recent CHEST guidelines recommending a therapeutic trial of gabapentin for unexplained chronic cough after discussion about risks-benefit profile with the patients.[88] Other neuromodulators have also been studied, including amitriptyline[89] and pregabalin[90] (**Table 3**). Furthermore, more clinical trials are underway targeting

Table 3
Treatment options for functional laryngeal disorder

Medication	Type of Study (Number of Patients)	Dosage of Medication	Response Rate (%)
Gabapentin	RCT (primary symptom cough, N = 62)	Up to 1800 mg/d	74[87]
	Case series (primary symptom cough, N = 98)	100–900 mg/d	68[91]
Pregabalin	Cases series (laryngeal symptoms, N = 12)	75 mg BID, increased to 150 mg BID over 4 wk	83[90]
Amitriptyline	RCT (primary symptom cough, N = 28)	10 mg up to 100 mg at night	87[89]
	Case series (primary symptom cough, N = 18)	10 mg up to 40 mg at night	77[92]

Abbreviation: BID, twice daily.

specific neuronal receptors in both the peripheral and the central nervous systems (such as P2X3,[19] and TRPA1, TRPV4, and TRPA1).[15,20]

SUMMARY

A gold standard test for the diagnosis of extraesophageal GERD remains elusive. Laryngoscopy and EGD have poor predictive value for diagnosing GERD as the cause of laryngeal symptoms. Ambulatory pH-impedance monitoring and oropharyngeal pH monitoring are also limited and novel tests and biomarkers need further controlled trials before they can be recommended for diagnostic evaluation. The lack of a gold standard test for diagnosis, in addition to the variable response to PPI, has undoubtedly contributed to the economic burden of the disease in the United States. Antireflux surgery is recommended only in select cases. There are some promising new medical therapies focusing on neuronal hypersensitivity on the horizon.

DISCLOSURE

The authors have no relevant conflicts of interest pertaining to this article.

REFERENCES

1. El-Serag HB, Sweet S, Winchester CC, et al. Update on the epidemiology of gastro-oesophageal reflux disease: a systematic review. Gut 2014;63(6):871–80.
2. Patel DA, Harb AH, Vaezi MF. Oropharyngeal reflux monitoring and atypical gastroesophageal reflux disease. Curr Gastroenterol Rep 2016;18(3):1–7.
3. Francis DO, Rymer JA, Slaughter JC, et al. High economic burden of caring for patients with suspected extraesophageal reflux. Am J Gastroenterol 2013;108(6):905–11.
4. Sandler RS, Everhart JE, Donowitz M, et al. The burden of selected digestive diseases in the United States. Gastroenterology 2002;122(5):1500–11.
5. Everhart JE, Ruhl CE. Burden of digestive diseases in the united states part i: overall and upper gastrointestinal diseases. Gastroenterology 2009;136(2):376–86.
6. Koufman JA. The otolaryngologic manifestations of gastroesophageal reflux disease (GERD): a clinical investigation of 225 patients using ambulatory 24-hour pH monitoring and an experimental investigation of the role of acid and pepsin

in the development of laryngeal injury. Laryngoscope 1991;101(No4.Pt 2.-Suppl 53.-P):1–78.

7. Francis DO, Vaezi MF. Should the reflex be reflux? throat symptoms and alternative explanations. Clin Gastroenterol Hepatol 2015;13(9):1560–6.

8. Cherry J, Margulies SI. Contact ulcer of the larynx. Laryngoscope 1968;78: 1937–40.

9. Wright RA, Miller SA, Corsello BF. Acid-induced esophagobronchial-cardiac reflexes in humans. Gastroenterology 1990. https://doi.org/10.1016/0016-5085(90)91231-T.

10. Vaezi MF, Hicks DM, Abelson TI, et al. Laryngeal signs and symptoms and gastroesophageal reflux disease (GERD): a critical assessment of cause and effect association. Clin Gastroenterol Hepatol 2003;1(5):333–44.

11. Smith JA, Decalmer S, Kelsall A, et al. Acoustic cough-reflux associations in chronic cough: potential triggers and mechanisms. Gastroenterology 2010; 139(3):754–62.

12. Decalmer S, Stovold R, Houghton LA, et al. Chronic cough: relationship between microaspiration, gastroesophageal reflux, and cough frequency. Chest 2012; 142(4):958–64.

13. Herregods TVK, Pauwels A, Jafari J, et al. Determinants of reflux-induced chronic cough. Gut 2017;66(12):2057–62.

14. Wang AM, Wang G, Huang N, et al. Association between laryngopharyngeal reflux disease and autonomic nerve dysfunction. Eur Arch Otorhinolaryngol 2019; 276(8):2283–7.

15. Smith JA, Woodcock A. Chronic cough. N Engl J Med 2016;375(16):1544–51.

16. Hilton ECY, Baverel PG, Woodcock A, et al. Pharmacodynamic modeling of cough responses to capsaicin inhalation calls into question the utility of the C5 end point. J Allergy Clin Immunol 2013;132(4):847–55.e5.

17. McGarvey L, McKeagney P, Polley L, et al. Are there clinical features of a sensitized cough reflex? Pulm Pharmacol Ther 2009;22(2):59–64.

18. Hilton E, Marsden P, Thurston A, et al. Clinical features of the urge-to-cough in patients with chronic cough. Respir Med 2015;109(6):701–7.

19. Abdulqawi R, Dockry R, Holt K, et al. P2X3 receptor antagonist (AF-219) in refractory chronic cough: a randomised, double-blind, placebo-controlled phase 2 study. Lancet 2015;385(9974):1198–205.

20. Bonvini SJ, Birrell MA, Smith JA, et al. Targeting TRP channels for chronic cough: from bench to bedside. Naunyn Schmiedebergs Arch Pharmacol 2015;388(4): 401–20.

21. Vaezi MF, Katzka D, Zerbib F. Extraesophageal symptoms and diseases attributed to GERD: where is the pendulum swinging now? Clin Gastroenterol Hepatol 2018;16(7):1018–29.

22. Parsel SM, Wu EL, Riley CA, et al. Gastroesophageal and laryngopharyngeal reflux associated with laryngeal malignancy: a systematic review and meta-analysis. Clin Gastroenterol Hepatol 2019;17(7):1253–64.e5.

23. Patel DA, Blanco M, Vaezi MF. Laryngopharyngeal reflux and functional laryngeal disorder: perspective and common practice of the general gastroenterologist. Gastroenterol Hepatol (N Y) 2018;14(9):512–20.

24. Barry DW, Vaezi MF. Laryngopharyngeal reflux: more questions than answers. Cleve Clin J Med 2010. https://doi.org/10.3949/ccjm.77a.09121.

25. Branski RC, Bhattacharyya N, Shapiro J. The reliability of the assessment of endoscopic laryngeal findings associated with laryngopharyngeal reflux disease. Laryngoscope 2002;112(6):1019–24.

26. Hicks DM, Ours TM, Abelson TI, et al. The prevalence of hypopharynx findings associated with gastroesophageal reflux in normal volunteers. J Voice 2002; 16(4):564–79.

27. Milstein CF, Charbel S, Hicks DM, et al. Prevalence of laryngeal irritation signs associated with reflux in asymptomatic volunteers: impact of endoscopic technique (rigid vs. flexible laryngoscope). Laryngoscope 2005;115(12):2256–61.

28. Swoger J, Ponsky J, Hicks DM, et al. Surgical fundoplication in laryngopharyngeal reflux unresponsive to aggressive acid suppression: a controlled study. Clin Gastroenterol Hepatol 2006;4(4):433.e1.

29. Belafsky P, Postma G, Koufman JA. The validity and reliability of the reflux finding score. Laryngoscopy 2001;111:1313–7. Available at: https://pdfs.semanticscholar.org/7360/2a0e0828226bf82e4435a2eec06a609984a9.pdf.

30. Kelchner LN, Horne J, Lee L, et al. Reliability of speech-language pathologist and otolaryngologist ratings of laryngeal signs of reflux in an asymptomatic population using the reflux finding score. J Voice 2007;21(1):92–100.

31. Chang BA, MacNeil SD, Morrison MD, et al. The reliability of the reflux finding score among general otolaryngologists. J Voice 2015;29(5):572–7.

32. Rosen R, Mitchell PD, Amirault J, et al. The edematous and erythematous airway does not denote pathologic gastroesophageal reflux. J Pediatr 2017;183:127–31.

33. Zerbib F. The prevalence of oesophagitis in "silent" gastro-oesophageal reflux disease: higher than expected? Dig Liver Dis 2015;47(1):12–3.

34. Rafii B, Taliercio S, Achlatis S, et al. Incidence of underlying laryngeal pathology in patients initially diagnosed with laryngopharyngeal reflux. Laryngoscope 2014; 124:1420–4.

35. Fletcher KC, Goutte M, Slaughter JC, et al. Significance and degree of reflux in patients with primary extraesophageal symptoms. Laryngoscope 2011;121(12): 2561–5.

36. Gupta R, Sataloff RT. Laryngopharyngeal reflux: current concepts and questions. Curr Opin Otolaryngol Head Neck Surg 2009;17(3):143–8.

37. Kavitt RT, Higginbotham T, Slaughter JC, et al. Symptom reports are not reliable during ambulatory reflux monitoring. Am J Gastroenterol 2012;107(12):1826–32.

38. Vaezi MF, Schroeder PL, Richter JE. Reproducibility of proximal probe pH parameters in 24-hour ambulatory esophageal pH monitoring. Am J Gastroenterol 1997; 92(5):825–9.

39. Ahmed T, Vaezi MF. The role of pH monitoring in extraesophageal gastroesophageal reflux disease. Gastrointest Endosc Clin N Am 2005. https://doi.org/10.1016/j.giec.2004.10.006.

40. Joniau S, Bradshaw A, Esterman A, et al. Reflux and laryngitis: a systematic review. Otolaryngol Head Neck Surg 2007;136(5):686–92.

41. Sun G, Muddana S, Slaughter JC, et al. A new pH catheter for laryngopharyngeal reflux: normal values. Laryngoscope 2009;119(8):1639–43.

42. Wiener GJ, Tsukashima R, Kelly C, et al. Oropharyngeal pH monitoring for the detection of liquid and aerosolized supraesophageal gastric reflux. J Voice 2009;23(4):498–504.

43. Ayazi S, Lipham JC, Hagen JA, et al. A new technique for measurement of pharyngeal pH: normal values and discriminating pH threshold. J Gastrointest Surg 2009;13(8):1422–9.

44. Yuksel ES, Slaughter JC, Mukhtar N, et al. An oropharyngeal pH monitoring device to evaluate patients with chronic laryngitis. Neurogastroenterol Motil 2013; 25(5):315–23.

45. Andrews TM, Orobello N. Histologic versus pH probe results in pediatric laryng-opharyngeal reflux. Int J Pediatr Otorhinolaryngol 2013;77(5):813–6.
46. Chiou E, Rosen R, Jiang H, et al. Diagnosis of supra-esophageal gastric reflux: correlation of oropharyngeal pH with esophageal impedance monitoring for gastro-esophageal reflux. Neurogastroenterol Motil 2011;23(8). https://doi.org/10.1111/j.1365-2982.2011.01726.x.
47. Ummarino D, Vandermeulen L, Roosens B, et al. Gastroesophageal reflux evaluation in patients affected by chronic cough: restech versus multichannel intraluminal impedance/pH metry. Laryngoscope 2013;123(4):980–4.
48. Becker V, Graf S, Schlag C, et al. First agreement analysis and day-to-day comparison of pharyngeal pH monitoring with pH/impedance monitoring in patients with suspected laryngopharyngeal reflux. J Gastrointest Surg 2012;16(6):1096–101.
49. Chheda NN, Seybt MW, Schade RR, et al. Normal values for pharyngeal pH monitoring. Ann Otol Rhinol Laryngol 2009;118(3):166–71.
50. Yadlapati R, Pandolfino JE, Lidder AK, et al. Oropharyngeal pH testing does not predict response to proton pump inhibitor therapy in patients with laryngeal symptoms. Am J Gastroenterol 2016;111(11):1517–24.
51. Worrell SG, DeMeester SR, Greene CL, et al. Pharyngeal pH monitoring better predicts a successful outcome for extraesophageal reflux symptoms after antireflux surgery. Surg Endosc 2013;27(11):4113–8.
52. Vailati C, Mazzoleni G, Bondi S, et al. Oropharyngeal pH monitoring for laryngo-pharyngeal reflux: is it a reliable test before therapy? J Voice 2013;27(1):84–9.
53. Friedman M, Maley A, Kelley K, et al. Impact of pH monitoring on laryngopharyngeal reflux treatment: improved compliance and symptom resolution. Otolaryngol Head Neck Surg 2011;144(4):558–62.
54. Roman S, Gyawali CP, Savarino E, et al. Ambulatory reflux monitoring for diagnosis of gastro-esophageal reflux disease: update of the Porto consensus and recommendations from an international consensus group. Neurogastroenterol Motil 2017;29(10):1–15.
55. Bajbouj M, Becker V, Neuber M, et al. Combined pH-metry/impedance monitoring increases the diagnostic yield in patients with atypical gastroesophageal reflux symptoms. Digestion 2007;76(3–4):223–8.
56. Francis DO, Goutte M, Slaughter JC, et al. Traditional reflux parameters and not impedance monitoring predict outcome after fundoplication in extraesophageal reflux. Laryngoscope 2011;121(9):1902–9.
57. Kavitt RT, Yuksel ES, Slaughter JC, et al. The role of impedance monitoring in patients with extraesophageal symptoms. Laryngoscope 2013;123(10):2463–8.
58. Dhillon VK, Akst LM. How to approach laryngopharyngeal reflux: an otolaryngology perspective. Curr Gastroenterol Rep 2016;18(8). https://doi.org/10.1007/s11894-016-0515-z.
59. Barona-Lleo L, Barona-De Guzman R, Krstulovic C. The diagnostic usefullness of the salivary pepsin test in symptomatic laryngopharyngeal reflux. J Voice 2018. https://doi.org/10.1016/j.jvoice.2018.07.008.
60. Knight J, Lively MO, Johnston N, et al. Sensitive pepsin immunoassay for detection of laryngopharyngeal reflux. Laryngoscope 2005;115(8):1473–8.
61. Printza A, Speletas M, Triaridis S, et al. Is pepsin detected in the saliva of patients who experience pharyngeal reflux? Hippokratia 2007;11(3):145–9.
62. Calvo-Henríquez C, Ruano-Ravina A, Vaamonde P, et al. Is pepsin a reliable marker of laryngopharyngeal reflux? a systematic review. Otolaryngol Head Neck Surg 2017;157(3):385–91.

63. Hoppo T, Zaidi AH, Matsui D, et al. Sep70/Pepsin expression in hypopharynx combined with hypopharyngeal multichannel intraluminal impedance increases diagnostic sensitivity of laryngopharyngeal reflux. Surg Endosc 2018;32(5): 2434–41.

64. Wang J, Zhao Y, Ren J, et al. Pepsin in saliva as a diagnostic biomarker in laryngopharyngeal reflux: a meta-analysis. Eur Arch Otorhinolaryngol 2018;275(3): 671–8.

65. Komatsu Y, Kelly LA, Zaidi AH, et al. Hypopharyngeal pepsin and Sep70 as diagnostic markers of laryngopharyngeal reflux: preliminary study. Surg Endosc 2015; 29(5):1080–7.

66. Yadlapati R, Furuta GT, Wani S. The ratio of SEP70 to pepsin as a biomarker of laryngopharyngeal reflux. Gastroenterology 2018;155(1):224–6.

67. Ates F, Yuksel ES, Higginbotham T, et al. Mucosal impedance discriminates GERD from non-GERD conditions. Gastroenterology 2015;148(2):334–43.

68. Patel DA, Higginbotham T, Slaughter JC, et al. Development and validation of a mucosal impedance contour analysis system to distinguish esophageal disorders. Gastroenterology 2019;156(6):1617–26.e1.

69. Kavitt RT, Lal P, Yuksel ES, et al. Esophageal mucosal impedance pattern is distinct in patients with extraesophageal reflux symptoms and pathologic acid reflux. J Voice 2017;31(3):347–51.

70. Patel DA, Sharda R, Choksi YA, et al. Model to select on-therapy vs off-therapy tests for patients with refractory esophageal or extraesophageal symptoms. Gastroenterology 2018;155(6):1729–40.e1.

71. Karkos PD, Wilson JA. Empiric treatment of laryngopharyngeal reflux with proton pump inhibitors: a systematic review. Laryngoscope 2006;116(1):144–8.

72. Qadeer MA, Phillips CO, Lopez AR, et al. Proton pump inhibitor therapy for suspected GERD-related chronic laryngitis: a meta-analysis of randomized controlled trials. Am J Gastroenterol 2006;101(11):2646–54.

73. Huaiyuan G, Haijun M, Jinliang W. Proton pump inhibitor therapy for the treatment of laryngopharyngeal reflux. J Clin Gastroenterol 2015;50(4):1–6.

74. Spantideas N, Drosou E, Bougea A, et al. Proton pump inhibitors for the treatment of laryngopharyngeal reflux. a systematic review. J Voice 2019. https://doi.org/10. 1016/j.jvoice.2019.05.005.

75. Lechien JR, Saussez S, Schindler A, et al. Clinical outcomes of laryngopharyngeal reflux treatment: a systematic review and meta-analysis. Laryngoscope 2019; 129(5):1174–87.

76. Yoon YH, Park KW, Lee SH, et al. Efficacy of three proton-pump inhibitor therapeutic strategies on laryngopharyngeal reflux disease; a prospective randomized double-blind study. Clin Otolaryngol 2019;44(4):612–8.

77. Glicksman JT, Mick PT, Fung K, et al. Prokinetic agents and laryngopharyngeal reflux disease. Laryngoscope 2014;124(10):2375–9.

78. Li S, Shi S, Chen F, et al. The effects of baclofen for the treatment of gastroesophageal reflux disease: a meta-analysis of randomized controlled trials. Gastroenterol Res Pract 2014;2014. https://doi.org/10.1155/2014/307805.

79. Lee YC, Jung AR, Kwon OE, et al. The effect of baclofen combined with a proton pump inhibitor in patients with refractory laryngopharyngeal reflux: a prospective, open-label study in thirty-two patients. Clin Otolaryngol 2019;44(3):431–4.

80. Koufman JA. Low-acid diet for recalcitrant laryngopharyngeal reflux: therapeutic benefits and their implications. Ann Otol Rhinol Laryngol 2011;120(5):281–7.

81. Lechien JR, Finck C, Khalife M, et al. Change of signs, symptoms and voice quality evaluations throughout a 3- to 6-month empirical treatment for laryngopharyngeal reflux disease. Clin Otolaryngol 2018;43(5):1273–82.

82. Sidwa F, Moore AL, Alligood E, et al. Surgical treatment of extraesophageal manifestations of gastroesophageal reflux disease. World J Surg 2017;41(10):2566–71.

83. Lechien JR, Dapri G, Dequanter D, et al. Surgical treatment for laryngopharyngeal reflux disease: a systematic review. JAMA Otolaryngol Head Neck Surg 2019;145(7):655–66.

84. Shaker R, Babaei A, Naini SR. Prevention of esophagopharyngeal reflux by augmenting the upper esophageal sphincter pressure barrier. Laryngoscope 2014;124(10):2268–74.

85. Yadlapati R, Craft J, Adkins CJ, et al. The upper esophageal sphincter assist device is associated with symptom response in reflux-associated laryngeal symptoms. Clin Gastroenterol Hepatol 2018;16(10):1670–2.

86. Roman S, Keefer L, Imam H, et al. Majority of symptoms in esophageal reflux PPI non-responders are not related to reflux. Neurogastroenterol Motil 2015;27(11):1667–74.

87. Ryan NM, Birring SS, Gibson PG. Gabapentin for refractory chronic cough: a randomised, double-blind, placebo-controlled trial. Lancet 2012;380(9853):1583–9.

88. Gibson P, Wang G, McGarvey L, et al. Treatment of unexplained chronic cough chest guideline and expert panel report. Chest 2016;149(1):27–44.

89. Jeyakumar A, Brickman TM, Haben M. Effectiveness of amitriptyline versus cough suppressants in the treatment of chronic cough resulting from postviral vagal neuropathy. Laryngoscope 2006;116(12):2108–12.

90. Halum SL, Sycamore DL, McRae BR. A new treatment option for laryngeal sensory neuropathy. Laryngoscope 2009;119(9):1844–7.

91. Lee B, Woo P. Chronic cough as a sign of laryngeal sensory neuropathy: diagnosis and treatment. Ann Otol Rhinol Laryngol 2005;114(4):253–7.

92. Bastian ZJ, Bastian RW. The use of neuralgia medications to treat sensory neuropathic cough: our experience in a retrospective cohort of thirty-two patients. PeerJ 2015;3:e816.

Moving?

Make sure your subscription moves with you!

To notify us of your new address, find your **Clinics Account Number** (located on your mailing label above your name), and contact customer service at:

Email: journalscustomerservice-usa@elsevier.com

800-654-2452 (subscribers in the U.S. & Canada)
314-447-8871 (subscribers outside of the U.S. & Canada)

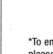

Fax number: 314-447-8029

Elsevier Health Sciences Division
Subscription Customer Service
3251 Riverport Lane
Maryland Heights, MO 63043

ELSEVIER

Printed and bound by CPI Group (UK) Ltd, Croydon, CR0 4YY

08/05/2025

01864691-0009